Trauma Surgery

Handbooks in General Surgery

W0043373

Kirby I. Bland • Michael G. Sarr
Markus W. Büchler • Attila Csendes
Oliver James Garden • John Wong
Editors

Trauma Surgery

Handbooks in General Surgery

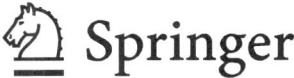 Springer

Editors

Kirby I. Bland, MD
Fay Fletcher Kerner Professor
and Chairman
Department of Surgery
Deputy Director,
Comprehensive Cancer Center
University of Alabama School
of Medicine
Birmingham, AL, USA

Markus W. Büchler, MD
Professor of Surgery and
Chairman
Department of General
and Visceral Surgery
University of Heidelberg
Heidelberg, Germany

Attila Csendes, MD, FACS
(Hon)
Professor of Surgery and
Chairman
Department of Surgery
University Hospital
Santiago, Chile

Michael G. Sarr, MD
James C. Mason Professor
of Surgery
Department of Surgery
Mayo Clinic College of
Medicine
Rochester, MN, USA

O. James Garden, MBChB, MD,
FRCS (Ed), FRCP (Ed),
FRACS (Hon)
Regius Professor of Clinical
Surgery
Department of Clinical and
Surgical Sciences
The University of Edinburgh
Royal Infirmary of Edinburgh
Edinburgh, UK

John Wong, BSc (Med (Syd)),
MBBS
(Syd), PhD (Syd), MD (Hon
(Syd)), FRACS, FRCS (Edin),
FRCS (Glasg), FACS (Hon)
Chair Professor
Department of Surgery
The University of Hong Kong
Queen Mary Hospital
Hong Kong, China

ISBN 978-1-84996-374-9   e-ISBN 978-1-84996-375-6

DOI 10.1007/978-1-84996-375-6

Springer London Dordrecht Heidelberg New York

British Library Cataloguing in Publication Data

A catalogue record for this book is available from the British Library

Library of Congress Control Number: 2010937968

Springer is part of Springer Science+Business Media (www.springer.com)

Preface

The editors designed the original textbook, *General Surgery: Principles and International Practice*, from which this shorter paperback monograph on trauma surgery was taken to be an accessible, concise, and state-of-the-art volume that explores and documents evolutionary principles in the practice of surgery. This work is aimed at the general surgeon and the resident in training. The scientific community continues to witness extraordinary advances in the therapy of both benign and malignant surgical diseases of various organ sites. Much of this progress has been evident over the past decade with new concepts and techniques of management that allow the surgeon to integrate this discipline with medicine, pharmacology, immunology, biostatistics, pathology, genetics, medical and radiation oncology, and diagnostic radiology and imaging. Further, each of these major disciplines contributes a small component for the diagnostic and therapeutic approaches to clinical care; hence the comprehensive planning, integration, and provision of patient care throughout the preoperative, intraoperative, and postoperative phases of care remains essential in the successful practice of our specialty.

The editors acknowledge that the aim of this work is to provide an illustrative, instructive, and comprehensive review that depicts the rationale of basic operative principles essential to surgical therapy. In organizing this monograph, the editors chose authors renowned in the disciplines for illustrating, forming, and depicting in a comprehensive fashion the surgical therapy expectant for metabolic, infectious, endocrine, and neoplastic abnormalities in adult and pediatric patients **from a truly international and multi-continental perspective.** The editors and authors were chosen carefully from across geographies and also from multi-cultural and diverse locations. While the authors consider this text to be inclusive regarding the technical and operative conditions for perioperative care in this field, its purpose should not be intended to replace standard textbooks of surgery nor should it be considered complete in its coverage of pathophysiologic disorders. In contrast, this monograph is organized to familiarize practicing surgeons, residents, and fellows with state-of-the-art surgical principles and techniques essential to contemporary practice. Therefore, the tenor of this monograph on trauma surgery has been developed to coexist with other major surgical reference texts that are dedicated—some in more comprehensive fashion—to the therapy of individual organs of systemic diseases. This monograph is much more a "working text" for the practicing surgeon with emphasis on diagnosis and treatment of traumatic injury. Along with this monograph, nine other paperback monographs are available and focus on the general principles of surgery, critical care, esophagus and stomach, small bowel, colorectal, liver and biliary, pancreas and spleen, oncology, and endocrine organs, all adapted from the primary textbook— *General Surgery: International Principles and Practice.*

The chapters in this monograph on trauma surgery include a condensed bibliography of highly selective journal articles, reviews, and text. In this manner of attempting to be concise, we hope to provide a precise focus for the education of the reader relative to accepted surgical principles involved in patient care. Moreover, the editors have sought to provide a counterpoint view for the selection of therapy by presenting at the opening of each chapter a list of "Pearls and Pitfalls" that highlight particular concerns or controversies. The chapters provide pertinent, though not exhaustive, summaries of anatomy and physiology, a history of surgical illness, and stages of operative approaches with relevant technical considerations outlined in an easily understandable manner. Complications are reviewed when appropriate for the organ system, diseases, and problem. The text is supported amply by line drawings and photographs that depict anatomic or technical principles. The editors have made every attempt to minimize duplicative or repetitive discussions except when controversial or state-of-the-art issues are presented. Moreover, the editors have attempted to ensure that accurate presentations and illustrations depict properly the most complex problems confronted by the general surgeon.

Finally, in an attempt to address advances in contemporary concepts, the text has been organized to address in detail expeditious, safe, and anatomically accurate operations and incorporate standard as well as evolving surgical principles and techniques. These principles have been tested in the clinics of valid scientific knowledge and are well supported by the time-tested approaches that have been provided by practicing surgeons. The editors are excited to be able to respond to the challenge of developing a truly international text and are indeed hopeful that our readers will find this focused monograph on trauma surgery to be a repository of insight, useful, and timely information.

Kirby I. Bland
Michael G. Sarr
Markus W. Büchler
Attila Csendes
Oliver James Garden
John Wong

Contents

1   **Initial Evaluation of the Trauma Patient** 1
    Donald A. Reiff and Loring W. Rue III

2   **Blunt Abdominal Trauma** 19
    Ricardo Ferrada, Diego Rivera, and Paula Ferrada

3   **Penetrating Trauma: Neck, Thorax,
    and Abdomen** 33
    Kenneth D. Boffard

4   **Vascular Trauma: Life-threatening
    Thoracoabdominal Injuries
    and Limb-threatening Extremity Injuries** 49
    C. Clay Cothren and Ernest E. Moore

5   **Thermal Injury** 67
    Nora F. Nugent and David N. Herndon

6   **Closed Head Injury** 83
    Philip F. Stahel and Wade R. Smith

7   **Spinal Trauma** 103
    Fritz U. Niethard and Markus Weißkopf

8   **Abdominal Compartment Syndrome** 121
    Hanns-Peter Knaebel

9   **Neurologic Physiology: The Brain
    and Its Response to Injury**   137
    Mamerhi O. Okor and James M. Markert

10   **Pericardial Tamponade**   155
    Gary A. Vercruysse, S. Rob Todd,
    and Frederick A. Moore

Index..   167

Contributors

Kenneth D. Boffard, MB, Bch, FRCS, FRCS (Edin), FRCPS(Glas), FCS(SA), FACS
Professor and Clinical Head, Department of Surgery, Johannesburg Hospital, University of the Witwatersrand, Johannesburg, South Africa

C. Clay Cothren, MD, FACS
Director, Surgical Critical Care Fellowship, Department of Surgery, Denver Health Medical Center, Denver, CO, USA

Paula Ferrada, MD
General Surgery Resident, Department of General Surgery, Beth Israel Deaconess Medical Center, Harvard University, Boston, MA, USA

Ricardo Ferrada, MD, MPH, FACS
Professor, Department of Surgery, University of Valle, Cali, Colombia

David N. Herndon, MD
Jesse H. Jones Distinguished Chair in Burn Surgery, Department of Surgery, University of Texas Medical Branch, Galveston, TX, USA

Hanns-Peter Knaebel, MD, MBA
Executive Vice President, Marketing & Sales, Clinical Science, Aesculap AG, Tuttlingen, Germany

James M. Markert, MD, MPH
Professor and Director, Division of Neurosurgery,
Department of Surgery, University of Alabama
at Birmingham, Birmingham, AL, USA

Ernest E. Moore, MD, FACS
Chief of Surgery and Trauma Services, Denver Health
System, Vice Chair, Department of Surgery, University
of Colorado Health Sciences Center, Denver, CO, USA

Frederick A. Moore, MD, FACS, FCCM
Division Head, Surgical Critical Care and Acute Care
Surgery, Department of Surgery, Methodist Hospital,
Houston, TX, USA

Fritz U. Niethard, MD
Professor, Orthopädische Universitätsklinik, Klinikum der
Rheinisch-Westfälisch-Technischen Hochschule, Aachen,
Germany

Nora F. Nugent, MBBCh BAO MRCSI
Department of Plastic Surgery, Cork University Hospital,
Wilton, Cork, Ireland

Mamerhi O. Okor, MD
Assistant Professor, Division of Neurosurgery,
Department of Surgery, University of Alabama
at Birmingham, Birmingham, AL, USA

Donald A. Reiff, MD, FACS
Assistant Professor, Section of Trauma, Burns & Surgical
Critical Care, Department of Surgery, University
of Alabama at Birmingham, Birmingham, AL, USA

Diego Rivera, MD
Attending Surgeon
Hospital Universitario del Valle
Cali, Colombia

Loring W. Rue III, MD, FACS
Professor and Vice Chair Chief, Section of Trauma,
Burns & Surgical Critical Care, University of Alabama
at Birmingham, Birmingham, AL, USA

Wade R. Smith, MD
Director, Orthopaedic Trauma, University of Colorado
School of Medicine, Denver Health Medical Center,
Denver, CO, USA

Philip F. Stahel, MD
Associate Professor, Department of Orthopedic Surgery,
Denver Health Medical Center, University of Colorado
School of Medicine, Denver, CO, USA

S. Rob Todd, MD, FACS
Assistant Professor, Department of Surgery, Methodist
Hospital, Houston, TX, USA

Gary A. Vercruysse, MD
Assistant Professor of Surgery, Division of Trauma, Surgical,
Critical Care, & Burns, Grady Memorial Hospital, Atlanta,
GA, USA

Markus Weißkopf, MD
Head of Spine Center, Hospital of Orthopaedic Surgery,
Schwarzach, Schwarzach, Germany

1
Initial Evaluation of the Trauma Patient

Donald A. Reiff and Loring W. Rue III

Pearls and Pitfalls

- Based upon the mechanism of trauma, all possible injuries should be excluded through the pursuit of appropriate examinations and diagnostic studies to reduce the risk of unrecognized occult injury.
- Uncooperative and combative patients should be assumed hypoxic, under the influence of drugs and/or alcohol, or to have suffered significant head injury.
- When in doubt definitive control of the airway using an endotracheal tube is appropriate.
- Use an end-tidal carbon dioxide detection device, followed by auscultation, to determine adequate placement of the endotracheal tube.
- If the esophagus is inadvertently intubated while attempting airway control, leave the tube in place. This will protect the airway from gastric contents and eliminate the need for subsequent esophageal intubation.
- Large, persistent pleural air leaks may be caused by a disrupted mainstem bronchus. This injury will likely require a second tube thoracostomy, selective intubation of the uninjured bronchus by experienced personnel, and surgical repair.
- Proximal extremity injuries should have intravenous (IV) access obtained in the contralateral uninjured limb.

K.I. Bland et al. (eds.), *Trauma Surgery*,
DOI 10.1007/978-1-84996-375-6_1,
© Springer-Verlag London Limited 2011

- A worsening base deficit is likely caused by unrecognized blood loss or inadequate volume resuscitation.
- Following blunt trauma, maintain spine precautions until the possibility of injury has been ruled out; apply cervical spine protection devices to patients who arrive without them.
- Failure to follow the ABCs of the primary survey for the multiply injured patient may seriously jeopardize survival; initial attention should not be directed toward the most dramatically obvious injury such as a mangled extremity.
- Failure to expose and examine the entire patient including the axillae, back, and perineum.
- Failure to perform a rectal examination and vaginal examination when appropriate.
- Failure to identify early signs of shock which include tachycardia, falling pulse pressure, and poor capillary refill. Compensatory mechanisms can maintain a normal systolic pressure until > 20–30% of the blood volume is lost.
- Placement of a subclavian central line on the uninjured side of a patient with thoracic trauma.
- Normal spine radiographs do not ensure the absence of osseous, ligamentous, or spinal injury. These diagnostic studies should be followed by a physical examination and comprehensive neurologic assessment when the patient is not under the influence of intoxicating agents and allows a complete evaluation.
- Failure to obtain appropriate and adequate radiographs in a timely fashion.

Injury remains the leading cause of death for the first 4 decades of life and results in over 300,000 permanent disabilities each year. Federal data indicate that since 2003, expenses for trauma-related disorders exceed all other medical and surgical conditions in the USA. Often termed the "Golden Hour," outcomes for injured patients are enhanced by expeditious and appropriate surgical care rendered soon after injury. With the development of the Advanced Trauma Life Support (ATLS) protocols designed by the American College of Surgeons in 1978, a system for care of the acutely injured patient was developed, and using this template, physicians and surgeons have a guideline for rapidly evaluating and treating critically injured patients.

Initial Approach to the Injured Patient

Upon arrival of the injured patient to the resuscitation suite, a member of the trauma team should obtain the mechanism of injury and other pertinent clinical data in rapid and organized fashion. Simultaneously, the "primary survey," focusing on life-sustaining physiologic functions, is conducted while monitoring devices are placed on the patient. As the primary survey is underway, life-threatening injuries are treated when identified. Following completion of this initial survey, the "secondary survey," which consists of the traditional "head-to-toe" physical examination, is performed, radiographic studies are obtained, and a definitive management plan is formulated for the patient.

Primary Survey

Airway

The initial evaluation of the polytrauma patient begins with an assessment of airway adequacy. Signs of compromise should be sought in the primary survey and are usually evident by an injured patient's inability to communicate verbally. Alert and conversant patients who respond with a normal-sounding voice suggest no immediate problem with airway patency while those appearing agitated may be hypoxic or under the influence of alcohol and/or drugs, unable to protect their airways. Patients who are minimally responsive or obtunded may be hypercarbic, have suffered traumatic brain injury, or also may suffer from alcohol and/or drug intoxication.

A quick and effective technique to establish a patient's airway is the chin lift and jaw thrust maneuver, which is particularly helpful when the tongue is the obstructing agent. These actions displace the soft tissue anteriorly, opening the upper airway and allowing for air passage. Other techniques include the placement of an oropharyngeal or nasopharyngeal airway. Oropharyngeal airway should be restricted to obtunded patients as this device is not tolerated by awake patients. Nasopharyngeal airways are less likely to induce vomiting but should be avoided if facial or basilar skull fractures are suspected. While these maneuvers are temporarily effective in maintaining a patent airway, their use in the acutely injured patient is frequently suggestive of the need for definitive airway control.

All trauma patients are treated as "full stomachs" and a rapid-sequence method for intubation is recommended. This technique begins with pre-oxygenation of the patient while the induction and paralytic agents are being administered. Yankour suction should be available to clear the oropharynx and supraglottic region of all secretions. Instruments necessary for a surgical airway should be available in the event that intubation is unsuccessful. Properly applied cricoid pressure will minimize the risk of aspirating regurgitated gastric contents during mask ventilation. While maintaining inline cervical stabilization and under direct laryngoscopic or bronchoscopic visualization, the cuff of the endotracheal tube is positioned distal to the vocal cords. Correct placement of the endotracheal tube is confirmed using an end tidal carbon dioxide detection device, auscultation of the chest, and a chest radiograph.

If attempts at intubation fail or the oral and nasal routes are contraindicated due to maxillofacial injuries or anatomic distortion, a surgical airway is mandated. The surgical cricothyroidotomy remains the preferred technique in these emergency situations. The authors' preferred method for creating a cricothyroidotomy is using a modified Seldinger technique. A vertical skin incision is centered over the cricothyroid membrane, which is then sharply opened horizontally using the scalpel. A flexible bougie tube is passed through the cricothyroidotomy into the trachea acting as the guide over which a #6 shiley or 7–0 endotracheal tube is advanced and secured.

Breathing/Ventilation

Once the airway is adequately addressed, oxygenation and ventilation must be ensured. Oxygenation can be assessed with the noninvasive pulse oximeter and confirmed with an arterial blood gas measurement. Satisfactory ventilation can be evaluated by inspection, palpation, percussion, and auscultation of the chest. If inadequate ventilation is detected, the airway should be reassessed to ensure that the esophagus has not been intubated inadvertently. If ventilation remains inadequate, life-threatening chest injuries that impede ventilation must be considered. These conditions include a tension pneumothorax, massive hemothorax, open pneumothorax, and flail chest.

A *tension pneumothorax* can result from either blunt or penetrating trauma to the lung, bronchi, or trachea, allowing air to continually leak into the pleural space. This differs from a simple pneumothorax in that the lung parenchymal injury remains patent and no chest wall defect is produced to allow venting of the progressively accumulating pleural air. Consequently, with each breath, the patient generates negative intrathoracic pressure, progressively accumulating air into the pleural space, resulting in collapse of the ipsilateral lung. The resultant increased pleural pressure will ultimately shift the mediastinum to the contralateral side. This mediastinal shift results in vena caval distortion, thereby decreasing venous return to the heart, resulting in depressed cardiac output and hemodynamic instability. Patients appear anxious with tachycardia, hypotension, marked respiratory distress, absent ipsilateral breath sounds, tracheal deviation to the contralateral side, and neck vein distention. Consequently, *tension pneumothorax* is a clinical diagnosis. It is quickly treated by placing a large bore angiocath into the second intercostal space aligned with the mid-clavicular line so as to decompress the pleural space. Definitive treatment requires the placement of a tube thoracostomy attached to 20 cm of water suction.

A *massive hemothorax* can occur as the consequence of either blunt or penetrating trauma due to an injury to an intercostal or hilar vessel. Massive hemothorax is defined as 1,500 cc of blood loss into the hemithorax with subsequent compression of the lung. The diagnosis is established when shock is identified in concert with absent breath sounds and dullness to percussion on one side of the chest. The injury is treated by simultaneous restoration of the intravascular space with crystalloids and blood products and decompression of the pleural space with a large (#38 or #40 French) tube thoracostomy. A chest radiograph should be obtained following placement of the chest tube to ensure that the hemothorax has been completely evacuated. Decompression of the hemothorax allows for the apposition of the parietal and visceral pleura, which frequently results in cessation of ongoing blood loss from the majority of pulmonary and osseous sources. If more than 1,500 cc of blood is initially evacuated or if blood loss exceeds 200 cc/h for the next 2–3 h, a thoracotomy may be required to surgically address ongoing hemorrhage.

An *open pneumothorax* or "sucking chest wound" results from a defect in the chest wall that exceeds two thirds of the diameter of the trachea. Following the injury, which is typically penetrating trauma, the intrathoracic pressure will equate with the atmospheric pressure. With each subsequent inspiratory effort, air will preferentially follow the path of least resistance through the thoracic defect and into the pleural space. The injury can be initially controlled with placement of an occlusive dressing over the wound and securing it on three sides. This creates a flap valve where air is permitted to escape from the pleural space during expiration but no air is allowed to enter during inspiration. Tube thoracostomy should be performed at a site remote from the injury. Frequently, definitive surgical closure of the chest wall defect is required.

A *flail chest* is defined as a fracture of three or more consecutive ribs in two or more places, with or without sternal involvement, allowing for paradoxical respiratory motion. Frequently, a flail chest will have an associated hemo- or pneumothorax and will require the placement of a chest tube. Although there is a severe disruption of normal chest wall movement associated with the flail segment, the resulting physiologic derangement is the consequence of the underlying pulmonary contusion and poor respiratory mechanics related to chest wall pain. Treatment is directed at providing physiologic support of the gas exchange abnormalities and alleviating pain.

Parenteral analgesics, particularly with patient-controlled analgesia, is the mainstay of therapy and should be employed liberally. Some patients benefit from early placement of thoracic epidural catheters. Thoracic epidural analgesia for flail chest has been demonstrated to improve the patient's maximum inspiratory effort, tidal volumes, and vital capacity. In the event pulmonary toilet and ventilation are still suboptimal with epidural analgesia, mechanical ventilatory support is required. Ventilator support is best implemented early, as this has been demonstrated to reduce overall duration of ventilatory support as well as mortality (Gianna et al., 1993).

Circulation

With the airway secured and ventilation deemed adequate, the circulatory system is the next priority. Shock is best defined as inadequate delivery of oxygen to meet the metabolic demands of peripheral tissue. The most common etiology of shock for the trauma patient remains hemorrhagic shock, but other sources including cardiogenic, compressive (cardiac tamponade or tension pneumothorax), and neurogenic (spinal injury) must be considered. Following blunt trauma, hypovolemic shock is most often due to intraperitoneal blood loss, pelvic fractures, musculoskeletal injuries, and/or thoracic trauma. Hemorrhagic shock associated with penetrating trauma can result from a laceration of any major blood vessel causing external exsanguination through the wound or internal exsanguination into any of the major corporal compartments.

The treatment of shock begins first with its recognition. The hallmark clinical signs of shock include tachycardia, hypotension, narrowing of the pulse pressure, cutaneous vasoconstriction, oliguria, and mental status changes to include the spectrum from apprehension to obtundation. Following the recognition of shock, initial management includes gaining access to the vascular system and staunching obvious external hemorrhage. IV access is obtained by placing two large-bore short angiocaths in peripheral veins. Once IV access is obtained, phlebotomy can be performed for basic laboratory studies and type and cross match. Initial volume expansion is achieved with a 2 l bolus of warmed lactated Ringer's solution. The volume required for the resuscitation of a patient is difficult to predict, but the "3 for 1 rule" can provide a rough approximation of a patient's initial fluid needs. This estimate assumes that a patient will need 3 cc of crystalloid for every cubic centimeter of blood loss. Patients in deep shock, or those who do not respond to their initial bolus of lactated Ringer should receive additional crystalloid boluses and early administration of blood products. The goal of any resuscitation strategy is reversal of the shock state and aggressive resuscitation should continue until adequate end organ perfusion and tissue oxygenation is achieved. Traditionally, the endpoints of shock resuscitation have been the restoration of normal blood pressure, heart rate, and adequate urinary output. Unfortunately, using these measures alone as a guide for adequate resuscitation may leave as many as 50–85% of trauma patients in "compensated" shock. In these situations, a patient's hemodynamic indices may be normal, but still have evidence of suboptimal tissue perfusion as demonstrated by the persistence of systemic acidemia, elevated lactate levels, and low mixed venous oxygen saturations. This situation can occur as blood flow and oxygen delivery is redistributed from the splanchnic bed to other critical organs such as the brain and heart. Recent resuscitation data suggest that in addition to restoring normal hemodynamic indices and urinary output, correction of the base deficit and restoring lactate levels to normal will result in significantly reduced mortality.

While fluid resuscitation is ongoing, the source of the circulatory collapse must be identified. Blood loss must first be excluded and may be as obvious as external hemorrhage or can occur occultly into any one or a combination of spaces to include the abdomen, thorax, retroperitoneum, or extremities. In the past, diagnostic peritoneal lavage (DPL) was the preferred technique used in the Emergency Department to exclude hemoperitoneum as a potential cause of hemodynamic instability. DPL remains a reliable study with reported sensitivities ranging from 90% to 96% and specificity from 99% to 100% (United States Medical Expenditures, 2003); however, this invasive and somewhat time-consuming procedure has been associated with nontherapeutic laparotomies. DPL will accurately identify hemoperitoneum but is unable to provide the source. Thus, a laparotomy is dictated for a solid organ injury that may have been better managed with nonoperative observation in an intensive care unit. In modern trauma centers, DPL's usefulness is limited because of readily available and rapid focused abdominal sonogram for trauma (FAST) and/or computerized tomography (CT) (Freedland et al., 1990).

FAST is a technique that surgeons can quickly master and is proving to be dependable, rapid, and noninvasive. The focused abdominal ultrasound is highly sensitive for detecting solid organ injury and is very reliable for identification of hemoperitoneum, with some studies demonstrating a sensitivity approaching 95% (Meyer et al., 1989). Its greatest value is realized in dealing with the hemodynamically unstable patient with multiple cavitary sources of potential blood loss. Ideally, efforts should be made to rapidly resuscitate and stabilize the patient in order to obtain a CT scan of the chest, abdomen, and pelvis, providing the clinician with definitive clinical information. Among patients in whom hemodynamic stability cannot be achieved and blood pressure liability precludes movement into an unsupervised setting such as the CT scanner, the FAST examination can quickly identify the presence or absence of a hemoperitoneum dictating the need for a laparotomy.

Pelvic fractures are an underappreciated source of blood loss in the polytrauma patient and blood loss can be of arterial, venous, and/or osseous origin. The patient can essentially exsanguinate from a pelvic fracture with the potential for several liters of blood to be sequestered in the retroperitoneum. Therapy begins with immobilization of the pelvis by applying a binder and/or providing surgical external fixation by an orthopedic specialist. This approach aligns the cancellous bone fragments and reduces the volume of the pelvis, thus allowing for a tamponade effect to arrest the venous and osseous hemorrhage. Failure to control hemorrhage in these circumstances is likely due to an arterial injury and may require angiography and therapeutic embolization. Femur fractures can be associated with 1,500 cc of blood loss and, similar to pelvic fractures, require immobilization as the initial treatment priority.

Neurologic Deficit/Exposure

The final aspect of the primary survey consists of identifying any gross neurologic deficit and exposing the patient completely. The Glasgow Coma Scale (GCS) is a detailed evaluation of function and an effective measure for evaluating the neurologic status of injured patients. The GCS is the sum of three components of assessment found in Table 1.1. Pupillary size, symmetry, and reaction to light are also assessed during the primary survey. These evaluations should occur early in the resuscitation process with frequent re-evaluations to document either patient improvement or deterioration. A worsening examination will prompt the need for additional therapy or diagnostic studies.

Among patients in whom brain injury is suspected with a concurrent depressed level of consciousness, steps should be taken urgently to definitively control the airway. Evidence supports that a single episode of hypoxemia is strongly associated with higher mortality and worse neurologic recovery. Similarly, a brief period of hypotension is correlated closely with poor long-term disability and worse mortality. Hyperventilation, previously employed for the head-injured patient, is currently contraindicated since it results in cerebral vasoconstriction and

TABLE 1.1. Glasgow coma scale.

Parameter	Score
Best motor response	
Normal	6
Localizes	5
Withdraws	4
Flexion	3
Extension	2
None	1
Best verbal response	
Oriented	5
Confused	4
Verbalizes	3
Vocalizes	2
None/Intubated	1
Eye opening	
Spontaneous	4
To command	3
To pain	2
None	1
Minor injury: 13–15	
Moderate injury: 9–12	
Severe injury: 8 or below	

decreased cerebral perfusion, thus potentially worsening brain injury. Current recommendations regarding ventilation support promote avoidance of excessive hyperventilation maintaining a $PaCO_2$ of 30–35 mmHg. This level of carbon dioxide balances cerebral blood flow and intracranial pressure. Hyperventilation is withheld exclusively for those with evidence of elevated intracranial pressure and impending herniation.

Completion of the primary survey requires that the patient be completely disrobed so that any obvious external injury is not overlooked. After logrolling the patient, the back, perineum, and axillae are examined and a rectal examination is performed. Afterwards, warm blankets are placed over the patient to minimize the risk of hypothermia. Other measures to preserve body temperature include heating the room, warming IV fluids and the inspired air in the ventilator circuit, and using environmental heaters such as the Bair Hugger. Hypothermia induces patient shivering to generate heat. This results in an increase in oxygen demand and worsening the shock state. Hypothermia can also impair both the primary and secondary hemostatic mechanisms.

Before beginning the secondary survey, the patient's clinical status should be reassessed by quickly reviewing all components of the primary survey with close attention to any alterations in vital signs and/or oxygen saturation. Additionally, basic radiographic and laboratory studies are performed. A minimum of three radiographic studies are performed for the trauma patient including an AP view of the chest and pelvis as well as a cross table lateral of the cervical spine. The information yielded from these studies is helpful in piecing together the clinical picture. Laboratory studies are frequently acquired when IV access is obtained. Additionally, an arterial blood gas should be drawn, usually from the femoral artery, to determine the extent of base deficit suggesting the degree of shock.

All severely injured patients should have a Foley catheter placed during their resuscitation. The only contraindication for Foley placement is a urethral injury which should be suspected with complex pelvic fractures, blood noted at the penile meatus, or a high-riding prostate detected during the rectal examination. If a urethral injury is suspected, a retrograde urethrogram is performed prior to the placement of the catheter.

A nasogastric (NG) tube is placed to decompress the stomach so as to reduce the risk of aspiration for intubated patients and those who are unable to protect their airways adequately due to CNS depression. Patients with midface instability or evidence of basilar skull fractures should have orogastric tubes placed instead of using the transnasal route to prevent potential iatrogenic injury.

Secondary Survey

The secondary survey consists of a review of the information regarding the injury mechanism, the patient's past medical history, and a complete "head to toe" physical examination. This portion of the evaluation should not begin until the primary survey has been completed, all life-saving interventions performed, and a satisfactory response to resuscitation observed. The physical examination needs to be performed in an organized and thorough manner beginning with the scalp and systematically moving caudally to the feet. Once completed, and based upon physical examination finding, the remainder of necessary diagnostic studies is obtained including radiographs of potential fractures, CT scans, and arteriograms.

CNS

As noted earlier, a brief neurologic examination is conducted during the primary survey. During the secondary survey, a more complete examination is performed evaluating the cranial nerves, motor strength of all extremities, spinal reflexes, and sensory losses to include pain, temperature, and proprioception from head to toe. Abnormalities identified in the physical examination should prompt further evaluation with a head CT or magnetic resonance imaging (MRI), as well as consultation with a neurosurgeon.

Blunt trauma patients should be assumed to have sustained a vertebral column injury until proven otherwise by an unequivocal physical examination and radiographic survey including CT imaging. Patients under the influence of alcohol and/or drugs and those with an abnormal GCS should remain in rigid cervical collars until their mental status has improved and a normal examination is demonstrated. The use of IV steroids in patients with spinal cord injury remains controversial. Current recommendations of a bolus followed by a continuous rate over a 23 h period are based upon a retrospective study demonstrating slight improvement in motor function of a single extremity in conjunction with steroid administration.

Currently, prospective studies are underway in an effort to clearly define the usefulness and exact role of steroids following acute spinal cord injury.

Head

Because of the abundant blood supply, lacerations of the scalp and face can bleed briskly and are usually controlled during the primary survey with direct pressure or quick placement of temporary sutures. During the secondary survey, these injuries should be debrided, adequately cleansed with a surgical soap, and primarily closed. Extraocular motion should be assessed and the face should be closely examined for any asymmetry. Most facial fractures can be detected by palpation of the bony prominences while fractures of the midface can be detected by inserting a finger into the mouth examining for instability of the hard palate or incisors. Maxillary or mandibular fractures are suggested by malocclusion. The tympanic membranes and external auditory canals are inspected with an otoscope. The presence of a hemotympanum or cerebrospinal fluid otorrhea is diagnostic of a basilar skull fracture. Further evidence of a basilar skull fracture is suggested by bruising around the eyes and behind the ears, the so-called "Battle sign". If facial or basilar skull fractures are suspected, a CT scan of the face should be performed to confirm the diagnosis and better define the injury.

Neck

The neck is typically divided into three zones. Zone I extends from the clavicles to the base of the cricoid cartilage, zone II extends from the cricoid to the angle of the mandible, and zone III spans the region from the angle of the mandible to the base of the skull. These zones are of particular importance in managing the patient with penetrating trauma. Unstable patients require surgical exploration. Hemodynamically stable patients with penetrating injury to zone I or III, because of the inherent anatomic inaccessibility, are best approached with a diagnostic evaluation which may include arteriography, bronchoscopy, rigid esophagoscopy, and a barium swallow. A great deal of debate continues regarding management of zone II injuries, with some authors advocating diagnostic evaluation as with zone I and III injuries. Alternatively, because of the ease of accessibility and exposure, as well as the high incidence of serious injuries in this unprotected region, patients with wounds that penetrate the platysma often undergo surgical exploration.

Chest

The chest should be reevaluated in the secondary survey by inspection, palpation, percussion, and auscultation. The chest radiograph should be closely examined for rib fractures, soft tissue injury, pneumothorax, hemothorax, subcutaneous emphysema, deviation of the trachea or esophagus, and shifted or widened mediastinum. Following blunt trauma, the diagnosis of a diaphragmatic rupture is suggested by an elevated left hemidiaphragm, loculated hemopneumothorax, or visualization of the NG tube in the left hemithorax.

A transected thoracic aorta is commonly associated with deceleration injuries and is frequently fatal at the scene. Clinicians having a high index of suspicion based upon the mechanism of injury and appreciating the hallmark signs seen on chest radiographs can identify these injuries early in the resuscitation. Radiographic findings consistent with a transected aorta include a mediastinal width greater than 8 cm, fracture of the first or second rib, obliteration of the aortic knob, deviation of trachea and esophagus to the right, pleural cap, elevation and rightward shift of the right mainstem bronchus, and depression of the left mainstem bronchus. Suspicion of injury should lead to a helical CT of the chest with IV contrast. These new generation scanners are proving to be effective at identifying aortic injury accurately with few missed injuries (Porter and Ivatury, 1998). Timing of surgery is dependent upon the patient's overall condition. Patients with hemodynamic instability require immediate surgery while stable patients can be medically optimized in the intensive care unit prior to surgical repair.

Abdomen

The abdomen encompasses the pelvis, the retroperitoneum, and the peritoneal cavity. During the secondary survey, a thorough examination of the abdomen is conducted using the traditional approach of inspection, palpation, and percussion. Visual examination of the abdomen should reveal any penetrating injuries, lacerations, or contusions. The flank and back are examined during the exposure portion of the primary survey when the patient is carefully log rolled. The abdominal examination is completed by rocking the pelvis to assess for instability and pain. Among patients for whom an acute laparotomy is not indicated based upon physical examination alone, CT imaging of the chest, abdomen, and pelvis should be undertaken.

Penetrating injuries to the abdomen deserve special attention. It should be remembered that the diaphragm ascends to the level of the fourth intercostal space and thus any penetrating injury affecting the lower chest wall can potentially injure the intra-abdominal viscera. All gunshot wounds to the abdomen and lower chest should be explored. Stab wound to the anterior abdominal wall should be explored locally for the presence or absence of fascial penetration. If exploration reveals that the posterior fascia has been violated or if the exploration is indeterminate, patients should undergo exploratory celiotomy. Penetrating wounds to the flank have the potential to cause occult intraabdominal injury and mandate, at a minimum, evaluation with a triple contrast CT study and serial examinations.

Extremities

The extremities should be examined for obvious fractures and lacerations. Suspected fractures should be radiographed and obvious fractures splinted as soon as possible. Assessment of the neurovascular status is of paramount importance. Hard signs of vascular trauma include active hemorrhage, distal pulse deficit, distal ischemia, and large or expanding hematomas. Among patients suffering fractures as a result of blunt force, persistent pulse discrepancies or hard signs following reduction of the fracture in the emergency department should prompt additional studies to eliminate the presence of a vascular injury. Patients with penetrating injury to an extremity should be carefully evaluated for the presence or absence of a hard sign of vascular injury and, if detected, surgical exploration is mandated (McKenney et al., 1996). Penetrating trauma in proximity to the major blood vessel without the "hard signs" is associated with a very low likelihood of significant vascular injury. Calculating an ankle/brachial index or performing color flow Doppler imaging and/or arteriography can be pursued. Prospective studies, however, have demonstrated that a thorough examination documenting the lack of "hard signs" of vascular injury is equally as sensitive as these diagnostic studies in determining the presence or absence of significant vascular injury. Motor or sensory deficits found on physical examination can result from either spinal cord injury, local peripheral nerve injury, or vascular injury with ischemia. Once vascular injury is excluded and the likely source of neurologic impairment is identified, appropriate consultation should be obtained.

Summary

A rapid and complete primary survey with early correction of life-threatening injuries has been shown to enhance patient survival and improve eventual outcomes. Delayed or inadequate resuscitation and unrecognized injuries ultimately will increase the patient's chance of developing multisystem organ dysfunction. Physicians who care for the acutely injured patient need to rehearse the steps of the primary and secondary survey until they become second nature to ensure that the "Golden Hour" is preserved and patient outcomes are enhanced.

Selected Readings

Boulanger BR, McLellan BA, et al. (1999) Prospective evidence of the superiority of a sonography-based algorithm in the assessment of blunt abdominal injury. J Trauma 47:632

Freedland M, Wilson RF, et al. (1990) The management of flail chest injury: factors affecting outcome. J Trauma 30:1460–1468

Frykberg ER, Dennis JW, et al. (1991) The reliability of physical examination in the evaluation of penetrating extremity trauma for vascular injury: results at one year. J Trauma 31:502–511

Gianna S, Waxman K, et al. (1993) Orotracheal intubation in trauma patients with cervical fractures. Arch Surg 128:903–906

McKenney MG, Martin L, et al. (1996) 1,000 consecutive ultrasounds for blunt abdominal trauma. J Trauma 40:607–612

Melton SM, Kerby JD, et al. (2004) The evolution of chest computed tomography for the definitive diagnosis of blunt aortic injury: a single-center experience. J Trauma 56:243–250

Meyer DM, Thal ER, et al. (1989) Evaluation of computed tomography and diagnostic peritoneal lavage in blunt abdominal trauma. J Trauma 29:1168–1170

Porter JM, Ivatury RR (1998) In search of the optimal end points of resuscitation in trauma patients: a review. J Trauma 44:908–914

United States Medical Expenditures (2003) United States Department of Health and Human Services – Agency for Healthcare Research and Quality. http://meps.ahrqgov/CompendiumTables/TC_TOC.htm

2
Blunt Abdominal Trauma

Ricardo Ferrada, Diego Rivera, and Paula Ferrada

Pearls and Pitfalls

- Patients suffering a high-energy trauma have solid viscera rupture in the abdomen and/or aortic rupture in the thorax until proven otherwise.
- Initial abdominal examination is inaccurate for detecting visceral injury, and especially so if the patient is in an altered mental state (alcohol, drugs, closed head trauma), pregnant, or paralyzed.
- Significant blunt abdominal trauma alone represents an indication for abdominal imaging.
- Fracture of the lower ribs ("abdominal ribs") should raise a very high suspicion of intraabdominal injury.
- Do not forget the possibility of hollow organ injury, especially with deceleration forces or a potential seat belt injury.
- An "elevated" left hemidiaphragm or a left "hydro/hemothorax" must raise the possibility of diaphragmatic rupture.
- The ultrasonographic focused abdominal sonography for trauma (FAST) exam has replaced virtually the diagnostic peritoneal lavage because of its ease, speed, sensitivity, and ability to be repeated easily.
- Computed tomography (CT) is a reliable imaging modality for solid organ and pelvic injury but requires a patient with stable vital signs.

K.I. Bland et al. (eds.), *Trauma Surgery*,
DOI 10.1007/978-1-84996-375-6_2,
© Springer-Verlag London Limited 2011

- Diagnostic peritoneal lavage (DPL) has essentially been replaced by the FAST, but DPL has some use when other tests are equivocal or when hollow organ injury is suspected.

General Considerations

Blunt abdominal trauma can be produced not only by direct contusion to the abdomen but also by deceleration injury or falls. Serious, devastating intra-abdominal injuries may be present despite the absence of external signs of trauma. This understanding underscores the importance of a complete evaluation in patients suffering high-energy trauma (Table 2.1), including a thorough physical examination, the judicious use of diagnostic modalities, and careful follow-up. The physical examination is a crucial part of the initial evaluation; however, signs of clinically important blunt abdominal trauma are not reliable in severe trauma. Physical examination alone has a sensitivity of only ~35%, positive predictive value of 30–50%, and a negative predictive value of about 60%. If the Glasgow Coma Score is less than 7, the sensitivity of the physical examination is only 20%. Other circumstances in which the physical examination is unreliable include alcohol or drug intoxication, spinal cord injury, pregnancy, and multiple extra-abdominal injuries (Table 2.2). Therefore, further investigation of the patient subjected to forces sufficient to have caused injury are necessary beyond just the physical examination,

TABLE 2.1. High-energy trauma.

Fall from higher than 10 ft

Ejection from a vehicle

Motor vehicle crash at speeds exceeding 45 miles/h

Motorbike accident

Major fracture

First rib fracture

Lower costal rib fracture

Seat belt restraint mark

TABLE 2.2. Unreliable physical examination.

Alcohol or drug intoxication

Spinal cord injury

Pregnancy

Glasgow coma score <10

Multiple extra-abdominal injuries

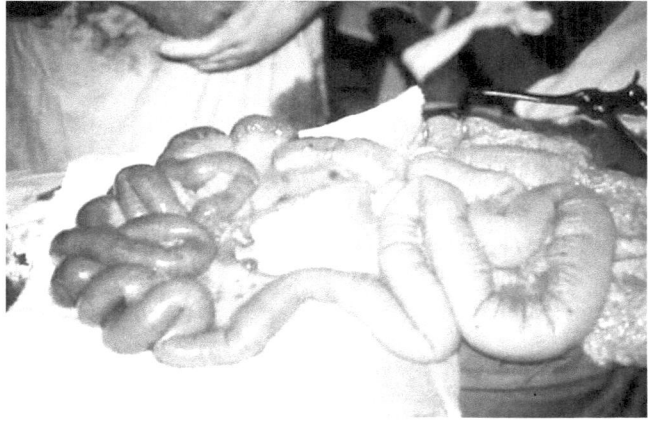

FIGURE 2.1. Mesenteric rupture due to a blunt abdominal trauma with subtle signs. The bowel was ischemic and had to be resected.

and the traumatologist must maintain a high index of suspicion of underlying intra-abdominal and intrathoracic injury.

In patients with lower rib fractures, called the "abdominal ribs," solid organ trauma should be suspected until proven otherwise. Splenic and/or hepatic injury is identified in 10–20%. As many as 40% of patients with hemoperitoneum show no findings on initial physical examination. For these reasons, the physical examination must be repeated serially by the same examiner, and consideration always given to diagnostic imaging (Fig. 2.1).

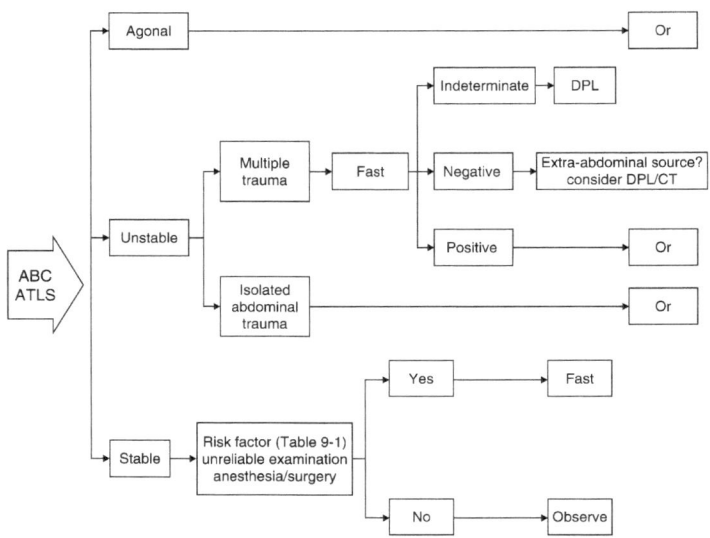

FIGURE 2.2. Algorithm for initial management.

The most frequently injured organ as a result of blunt abdominal trauma is the spleen (40–55%), followed by the liver (35–40%). Although the hollow organs are injured less frequently (15%), delay in diagnosis results in high rates of morbidity and mortality with these injuries. The added difficulty in diagnosis of hollow organ injury on physical examination alone adds further complexity to management (Fig. 2.2).

Diagnostic Procedures

Defining the extent of injury after blunt abdominal trauma can be difficult even for an experienced surgeon without the aid of diagnostic procedures. In most cases, significant blunt abdominal trauma alone is an indication for a more thorough evaluation, including at least some imaging modality.

Radiography

Chest x-ray must be a standard part of the initial evaluation of patients sustaining potential blunt abdominal trauma. Concomitant thoracic visceral injuries may occur and must be considered as well. Signs of abdominal visceral or diaphragm rupture are rarely seen on x-ray, but an elevated hemidiaphragm, an air/fluid level in the chest, or other findings suggesting the presence of intra-abdominal viscera in the chest require investigation or celiotomy. Although a rare finding, pneumoperitoneum may indicate hollow viscus injury warranting laparotomy. Just as with the physical examination, the abdominal x-ray can be unreliable in underlying intra-abdominal injury. Nevertheless, review of the abdominal part of a pelvic x-ray screening for pelvic fracture is of potential use, especially in the patient who is unreliable.

Ultrasonography

In 1992, Tso and colleagues evaluated the use of ultrasonography (US) in 63 patients with blunt abdominal trauma. This preliminary study demonstrated a sensitivity of 69%, specificity of 99%, and accuracy rate of 96%, similar to CT and diagnostic peritoneal lavage (DPL) at the same institution. Rozycki and colleagues reported their outcomes subsequently and coined the term focused abdominal sonography for trauma (FAST) in 1,540 patients (1,227 with blunt injuries and 313 with penetrating injuries). With an overall sensitivity of 84% and a specificity of 99%, US was most sensitive and specific for the evaluation of hypotensive patients with blunt abdominal trauma (sensitivity 100%, specificity 100%).

US has become the surgeon's and traumatologist's "stethoscope" for patients with abdominal trauma. The advantages of this technique are that it is relatively easy to learn, cost-effective, noninvasive, takes only a few minutes, has no radiation, can be repeated as many times as needed, and can be performed simultaneously with the resuscitation effort.

The goal of the FAST exam is to detect fluid in easily accessible areas: precordial (intrapericardial), Morrison's pouch, left upper quadrant pouch of Douglas, and the pelvis. The estimated number of examinations that a non-radiologist must perform to acquire acceptable accuracy ranges from 100 to 400 US exams. FAST can detect a volume of fluid as low as 200 ml; however, injuries not resulting in hemoperitoneum or hollow visceral injury without extravasation of enough enteric content may be missed. There are notable limitations of the FAST exam which include: operator dependency, increased difficulty in the obese or distended patient, the patient with ascites or subcutaneous emphysema, and poor ability to recognize solid parenchymal or hollow visceral injuries without substantial extravasation of enteric content. One major advantage is that the FAST exam can be repeated serially and when clinical status changes. In the absence of clinical instability, a negative FAST can allow ongoing evaluation and treatment of extra-abdominal injuries (Fig. 2.3).

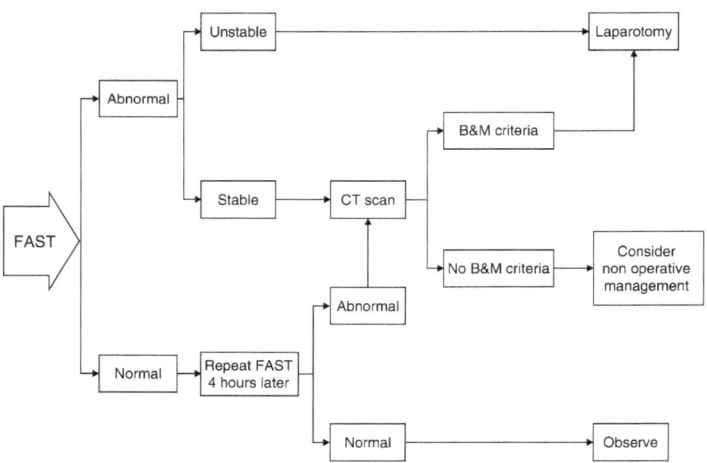

FIGURE 2.3. Algorithm for management according to the focused abdominal sonography for trauma (FAST) and computed tomography (CT) exam.

Computed Tomography

CT allows a complete and noninvasive assessment of the abdominal and pelvic cavities, retroperitoneal structures, soft tissues, and bones. CT is especially reliable for assessment of the liver and the spleen. In the kidney, CT allows assessment of not only the anatomy but the function as well. The accuracy in stable patients with blunt abdominal trauma is excellent, with a reported sensitivity and specificity approaching 98%. The negative predictive value is 99%, and thus a negative CT excludes very reliably the need for an immediate laparotomy in the vast majority of patients. For these reasons, CT has become the favored diagnostic procedure in blunt trauma, and should be obtained in most patients, provided they are hemodynamically stable.

CT is particularly useful when the physical examination is unreliable or equivocal or when nonoperative management is considered in the setting of stable patients with a positive DPL or FAST exam. Several additional advantages of CT are that it is noninvasive, can define the location and extent of solid organ or retroperitoneal injuries, can detect ongoing bleeding when intravenous (IV) contrast is used, and does not require hemoperitoneum, as do DPL and FAST exams. Unless contraindicated, IV contrast agent should be used when CT is obtained for evaluation of blunt abdominal trauma to examine renal function as to get a better definition of solid parenchymal injury, blood flow, and extravasation. Detection of hollow visceral injuries is less accurate and less reliable, even with quality contrast-enhanced CT. Nevertheless, certain findings on CT may suggest strongly the presence of an underlying injury to hollow viscera or to the mesentery; these CT findings include pneumoperitoneum, leak of the contrast agent into the peritoneal cavity, thickening of bowel wall or the mesentery, and free fluid without solid visceral injury. If any of these signs are found or there is other suspicion of hollow viscus injury, either DPL or an emergent laparotomy should be performed.

Diagnostic Peritoneal Lavage

Prior to the advent of the FAST exam, DPL had become the gold standard for blunt abdominal trauma. Only 30 ml of blood can produce a microscopically positive test. DPL is very sensitive (sometimes possibly too sensitive) and thus not specific. When negative, clinically important intra-abdominal bleeding is highly unlikely. In contrast, DPL is oversensitive in that not all patients with a positive DPL have a serious enough injury to warrant operative intervention. Additional limitations of DPL include the inability to detect retroperitoneal injury or solid organ injury in the absence of hemoperitoneum, and it is contraindicated in advanced pregnancy or with a history of multiple previous laparotomies; a pelvic fracture can produce a false-positive exam in the absence of solid or hollow visceral injury. The indications for DPL are similar to those for CT. Currently, with the FAST exam, DPL is used only rarely unless FAST is either unavailable or equivocal or when CT is contraindicated.

Prior to performing a DPL, a nasogastric (NG) tube and urinary catheter must be inserted. The technique may be performed open or with a needle and wire passed into the intraperitoneal cavity using the Seldinger technique. Under local anesthesia, an incision midline below the umbilicus incision is performed. When a pelvic trauma is suspected or confirmed, the incision should be made above the umbilicus in order to avoid entering a potention pelvic hematoma. Once the skin and the fascia are incised, the wire and catheter are inserted, removing this wire as the peritoneum is penetrated, and the catheter is advanced toward the pelvis. If the technique is open, the peritoneum should be incised under direct visualization. After the catheter is inserted, aspiration with a 20 ml syringe is performed. If more than 10 ml of gross blood is obtained, the test is considered positive and terminated. Otherwise, 1,000 ml of 0.9% normal saline is instilled into the peritoneal cavity, the patient is turned gently from side to side if possible, and the fluid is drained by gravity. The DPL is considered positive when the return fluid is grossly bloody or evidence of enteric content is seen. If the

TABLE 2.3. DPL interpretation.

Positive	RBC more than 100,000 mm³
	WBC more than 500/mm³
	Bile
	Bacteria
	Feces/intestinal content
Intermediate	RBC 50,000–100,000/mm³
	WBC 100–500/mm³

fluid is pink or clear, a sample is sent to the laboratory for quantitative determination of red and white blood cells or signs; the criteria are outlined in Table 2.3.

Initial Management

For practical purposes, we classify trauma patients according to hemodynamic status as moribund (agonal), unstable, or stable.

Moribund or Agonal Patients

Moribund patients are those with no spontaneous ventilatory effort, no femoral pulse, and no response to painful stimuli. These patients require an emergent airway and strong consideration of immediate operative intervention for suspected hemorrhage. Accordingly, after assuring airway and breathing (the A and B of the ABCs of resuscitation), a laparotomy and/or a thoracotomy must be considered. Whether a resuscitative thoracotomy prior to laparotomy improves the survival rate of these patients is controversial. Some authors have recommended clamping of the thoracic aortic, even in the emergency room setting, prior to laparotomy (in the operating room) in patients with refractory hypotension and abdominal distension secondary to massive hemoperitoneum. The rationale for this approach is to increase upper torso and intracranial blood pressure immediately and to prevent cardiac arrest after release of abdominal wall tamponade during celiotomy. The mortality in this setting is exceedingly high, with very few survivors; many traumatologists do not believe in this approach. The patients are taken to an operating room immediately, placed supine, and the abdomen explored with other minimal maneuvers. During abdominal exploration, the finding of significant or ongoing intra-abdominal hemorrhage may require cross-clamping the aorta at the diaphragmatic hiatus if there had been no thoracotomy. The surgeon must pack and compress the bleeding area(s) and seek more stable conditions by infusing a large amount of IV fluid and blood. Most of these patients require a shortened procedure (so-called damage control) with transfer to a surgical critical care unit for stabilization and later definitive repair of the intraperitoneal injury if they survive.

Unstable Patients

Patients are considered unstable when any vital sign, such as pulse, ventilatory rate, or blood pressure, is significantly abnormal. The instability is produced by either respiratory compromise or hypovolemia, so the initial approach (the ABCs) must include the establishment of the airway, ventilation, and circulation with immediate control of any external bleeding and IV access. After the management of airway and breathing, the next step is fluid resuscitation with a warm, balanced salt solution. The authors start with a bolus of 1,500 ml in patients of 140 lb (70 kg) of weight. If a patient recovers skin color and the vital signs normalize, additional IV fluid is infused at a lower rate, according to the response in the pulse rate and amplitude and urine output. If stability is achieved, patients are managed according to the algorithm for stable patients. In contrast, if the vital signs do not recover or improve only temporarily with fluid resuscitation and blood transfusion, then ongoing hemorrhage should be suspected, and operative intervention may be indicated.

Stable Patients

Patients are judged to be stable when their vital signs are normal initially or when the vital signs return to normal after the initial IV bolus. A more detailed clinical history must then be obtained. Careful evaluation is necessary to define the extent of injury. The decision for continued observation or intervention is based on the mechanism of injury and findings on evaluation. The decision to treat by observation requires careful and repeated assessment. As the physical examination may not be reliable in a number of cases, serial examination will be crucial in decision making.

Subsequent Management after Initial Evaluation

The majority of patients with blunt abdominal trauma arrive with no clinical signs of abdominal trauma with the exception of pain and possibly abdominal wall ecchymosis. Management depends largely on the stability of the patient and findings of diagnostic procedures.

In the group of stable patients, several situations require special mention. Patients who appear stable but have risk factors for potential serious injury mandate particularly careful observation, because delayed clinical deterioration may occur (Table 2.1). Those who fell from more than 10 ft, were ejected from a vehicle, were involved in a motor vehicle crash of more than 45 miles/h, or were in a motorbike accident must be considered high-energy trauma. Subtle signs such as fracture of the first rib, abdominal wall ecchymosis from the seat belt ("seat belt sign"), or major fractures of long bones or pelvis also imply high-energy trauma and warrant close observation. Fractures of the lower "abdominal" ribs should suggest possible abdominal solid organ injury. In patients with a closed head injury, intoxication, drug abuse, or those who require neurosurgery or orthopedic surgery where the physical examination will be unreliable for several hours because of the anesthetic, some objective evaluation of the abdomen is necessary, such as a FAST exam, CT, or DPL. As noted previously, the FAST exam has become one of the most important tests in diagnosis of severe blunt abdominal trauma. When the first view is negative, if there are any doubts, the FAST can be repeated on multiple occasions.

A major advance in the last two decades has been the use of primary nonoperative management for solid viscera injury, as guided by initial imaging and clinical response. Good evidence suggests that nonoperative management in both children and adults is safe, and the results are better than with a laparotomy in selected cases. Appropriate candidates for nonoperative management are those without active bleeding from solid viscera injury without evidence of hollow viscus or mesenteric injury. Observation requires hemodynamically stable patients in whom ongoing evaluation and observation can be performed. Quality CT imaging, a monitored environment, and access to emergent intervention are required (Table 2.4).

In selected patients with isolated solid viscera injury in whom contrast extravasation is seen either during the arterial or venous phase of the CT, a transcatheter arterial embolization may be considered. In contrast, nonoperative management should be abandoned in adults when hemodynamic status cannot be maintained after two units of packed red cells during the initial management or four units in the first 48 h, or if the embolization does not stop the extravasation at angiography.

TABLE 2.4. Requirements for non-operative management.

Hemodynamically stable

Absence of peritonitis

Contrast-enhanced CT without evidence of active bleeding

Monitoring in an intensive care unit

Staff available for repeated observation

Operation room available 24 h

The success rate of nonoperative management is high for isolated hepatic injury, but is less in splenic and especially renal injury, and is dependent on the extent of parenchymal injury (e.g., grade of liver and splenic injury). Risk factors for failure of nonoperative management includes the need for transfusion and free fluid over 300 ml in the abdominal cavity.

Selected Readings

ACEP Clinical Policies Committee, Clinical Policies Subcommittee on Acute Blunt Abdominal Trauma (2004) Clinical policy: critical issues in the evaluation of adult patients presenting to the emergency department with acute blunt abdominal trauma. Ann Emerg Med 43:278–290

Blackbourne L, Soffer D, McKenney M, et al. (2004) Secondary ultrasound examination increases the sensitivity of the FAST exam in blunt trauma. J Trauma 57:934–938

Fang J, Wong Y, Lin B, et al. (2006) Usefulness of multidetector computed tomography for the initial assessment of blunt abdominal trauma patients. World J Surg 30:176–182

Ferrada R, Birolini D (1999) Penetrating abdominal trauma. Surg Clin N Am 79:1331–1356

Hoff WS, Holevar M, Nagy KK, et al. (2002) Practice management guidelines for the evaluation of blunt abdominal trauma: the EAST practice management guidelines group. J Trauma 53:602–615

Menegaux F, Tresallet C, Gosgnach M, et al. (2006) Diagnosis of bowel and mesenteric injuries in blunt abdominal trauma: a prospective study. Am J Emerg Med 24:19–24

Peitzman AB, Harbrecht BG, Rivera L, et al. (2005) Failure of observation of blunt splenic trauma in adults: variability in practice and adverse consequences. J Am Coll Surg 201:179–187

Rozycki G, Ballard R, Feliciano D, et al. (1998) Surgeon performed ultrasound for the assessment of truncal injuries. Lessons learned from 1540 patients. Ann Surg 228:557–567

Velmahos G, Toutouzas K, Radin R, et al. (2003) Nonoperative treatment of blunt injury to solid abdominal organs. A prospective study. Arch Surg 138:844–851

3
Penetrating Trauma: Neck, Thorax, and Abdomen

Kenneth D. Boffard

Pearls and Pitfalls

Neck

- Never probe a wound in the neck if it is not bleeding—direct digital control may be preferable if it is.
- Always expect the worst.
- Always intubate early—the tube can be removed later if not needed.
- Paralyzing agents for airway control invite disaster.
- Always aim for proximal control of blood vessels.

Thorax

- All penetrating injuries of the abdomen may enter the chest (and vice versa). Assessment and investigation should therefore include both cavities, and include X-rays of the chest and abdomen.
- If the injury affects both the thorax and abdomen, unless in extremis, deal with the abdomen first.
- Fluid resuscitation must be mild to moderate.
- A double-lumen endotracheal tube will allow selective deflation of one lung, which may improve access and the ability to repair the injury.
- An emergency room thoracotomy will not revive a dead patient.

K.I. Bland et al. (eds.), *Trauma Surgery*,
DOI 10.1007/978-1-84996-375-6_3,
© Springer-Verlag London Limited 2011

Abdomen

- Blood is not an irritant. Blood in the abdomen is not painful.
- Bowel sounds can still be present, even in the presence of significant visceral injury.
- If the injury penetrates the peritoneum or diaphragm, always assume that the penetration has caused damage on the "dark side."
- Be careful of underestimating the impending disaster of a distending abdomen in a shocked patient.
- All penetrating wounds come in pairs. If you find an entrance wound, there will be either an exit wound, or a missile left behind.
- Always use metal markers to mark penetrating wounds before X-ray. Marked wounds and missile fragments should correspond on the relevant X-rays and correlate with the suspected organ involved in the injury.
- With non-operative management, success is not predictable by grade of injury or computed tomography appearance, but only on physiological stability. In the presence of hemodynamic instability, prompt exploration of the abdomen becomes urgent.
- A negative laparotomy is better than a positive post-mortem.

Penetrating Injuries of the Neck

Introduction

The high density of critical vascular, aerodigestive, and neurologic structures within the neck makes the management of pene-trating injuries difficult and contributes to the morbidity and mortality seen in these patients. However, there is a morbidity rate associated with exploration, and recently the policy of aggressive investigation and conservative surgery (including non-operative management) has become more common.

Management Principles

Current management of penetrating cervical injuries depends on several factors.

Primary Survey

Patients with signs of significant neck injury and hemodynamic instability will require prompt exploration. However, initial assessment and management of the patient should be carried out according to ATLS principles.

The major initial concern in any patient with a penetrating neck wound is early control of the airway. Appropriate protective measures for possible cervical spine injury must be implemented. A characteristic of neck injuries is rapid airway distortion with obstruction due to edema and hematoma, and often difficult intubation. The key to management is early intubation. The route of intubation must be considered carefully in these patients since it may be complicated by distortion of anatomy, hematoma, dislodging of clots, laryngeal trauma, and a significant number of cervical spinal injuries. These patients should be intubated as soon as possible, with appropriate neck protection. The use of paralyzing agents in these patients is contra-indicated, since the airway may be held open only by the patient's use of muscles. Abolishing the use of muscles in such patients usually results in the immediate and total obstruction of the airway, and no visibility due to the presence of blood, may be catastrophic. Ideally, local anesthetic spray should be used with sedation, and an immediate cricothyroidotomy below the injury should be considered when necessary. Tracheostomy should be reserved as a planned procedure in the operating theatre.

Control of hemorrhage should be undertaken by direct pressure where possible. If the neck wound is not bleeding, do not probe or finger the wound as a clot maybe dislodged. If the wound is bleeding actively, then the hemorrhage can be controlled by direct digital pressure, or as a last resort, by a Foley catheter.

Secondary Survey

The injured area is often related to anatomical areas. The structures injured are those related to the particular anatomical areas (Fig. 3.1). The neck is divided into:

- Posterior triangle
  - Behind the posterior border of sternomastoid muscle

- Anterior triangle, which is divided into
  - Zone I

- The area below the cricoid cartilage
  - Zone II

  The area between the cricoid cartilage and the angle of the mandible
  - Zone III

The area above the angle of the mandible

Two immediate questions must be answered:

- Is the patient stable?
- Does the injury penetrate platysma?

If stable, the investigation can be based on index of suspicion, and anatomical probability of injury. Investigation will be based on the areas of the neck involved (Fig. 3.2).

Management

In principle, all structures should be controlled and then repaired primarily. Arteries in Zones I and III will require proximal and distal control and probable repair. Subclavian artery injury carries specific risks. The key is proximal control with good exposure. Ideally this can be achieved with trans-femoral balloon control, but failing this, proximal control with thoracotomy or sternotomy and division of the clavicle (rarely excision) may be required. Veins can generally be tied off. All aerodigestive structures in Zone II should be repaired primarily with suitable (preferably suction) drainage.

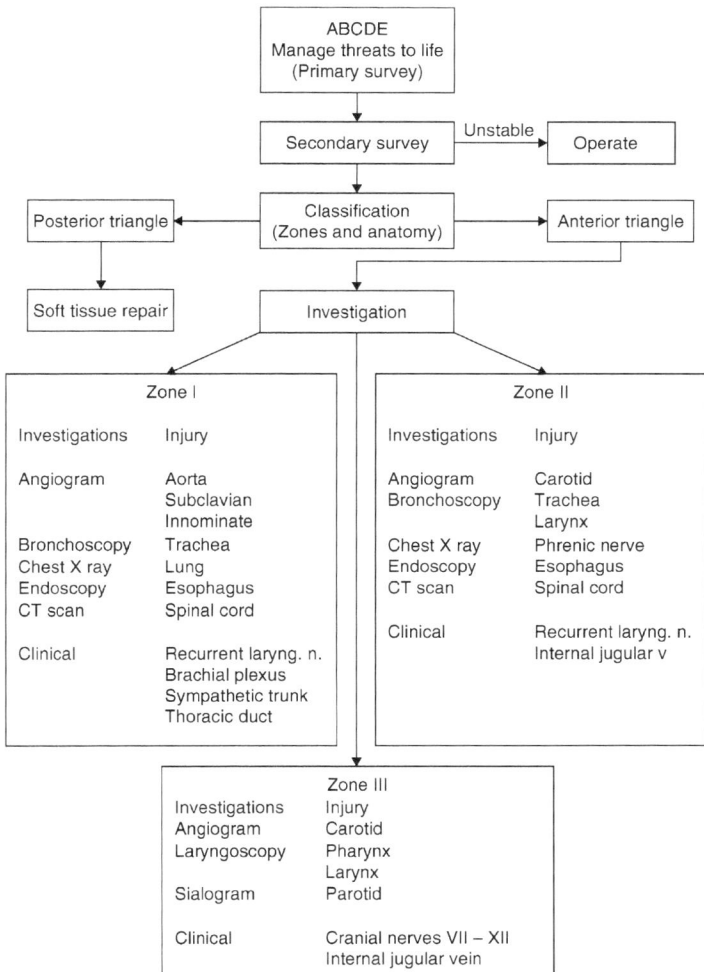

FIGURE 3.1. Investigation of penetrating injury to the anterior and posterior triangle of the neck.

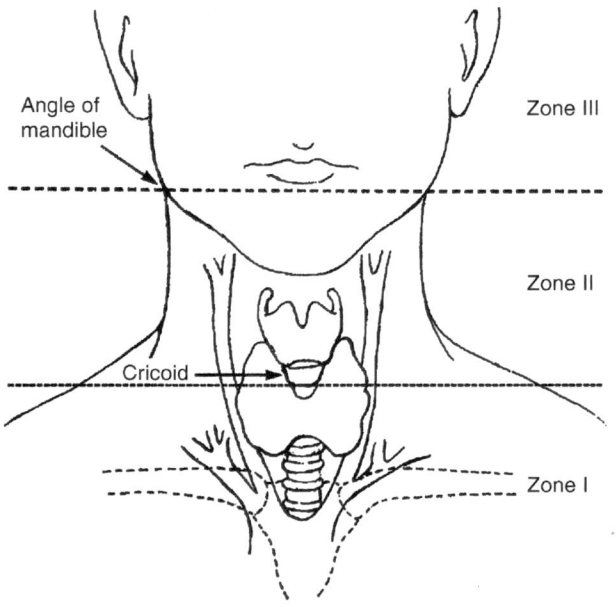

Figure 3.2. The anterior triangle of the neck showing the zones of the neck.

Penetrating Injuries to the Chest

It is best to artificially separate the "chest" and "abdomen" since there is a very high risk of injury to both cavities (Fig. 3.3). Each penetrating injury should be marked with a metal marker taped to the skin prior to radiography. This will give helpful information of the risks of individual organ involvement (Fig. 3.4).

Lethal injuries to the chest following penetrating injury include tension pneumothorax, massive bleeding (internally into the hemithorax, or externally), and cardiac tamponade.

Tension pneumothorax is diagnosed clinically with hypertympany on the side of the lesion, deviation of the trachea away from the lesion, and decreased breath sounds on the affected side. There is usually associated elevated jugular venous pressure in the neck veins. This is a clinical diagnosis,

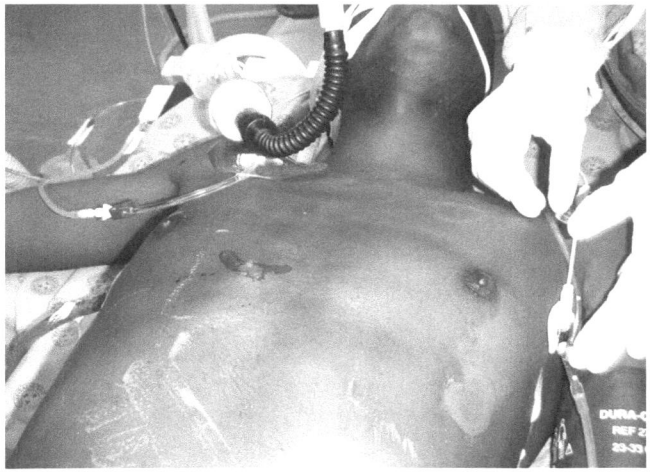

FIGURE 3.3. Patient with penetrating wound of the central torso.

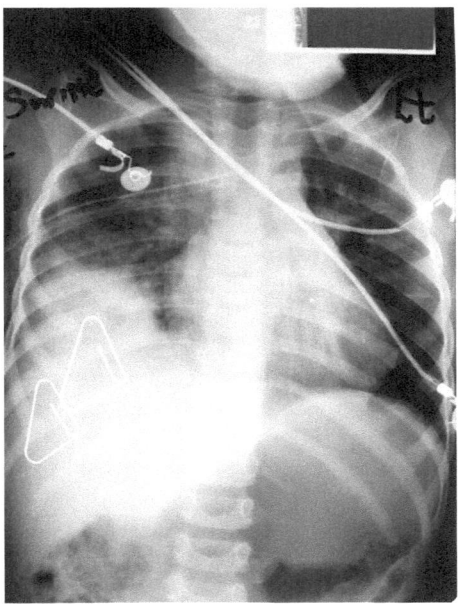

FIGURE 3.4. X-ray of chest showing metal markers.

and once made an immediate needle thoracostomy or tube thoracostomy should be performed to relieve the tension pneumothorax.

The diagnosis of cardiac tamponade frequently is difficult to make clinically. It is usually associated with hypotension and elevated jugular venous pressure. There are usually muffled heart sounds, that are difficult to hear in a noisy resuscitation suite. Placing a central venous pressure (CVP) line with resultant high venous pressures can confirm the diagnosis, although a low CVP in a shocked patient does not exclude tamponade. If ultrasound is available, this is an extremely helpful diagnostic adjunct. Once the diagnosis is made, if the patient is hypotensive, the tamponade needs to be relieved as soon as possible, since ultimately decompensation is sudden. Needle pericardiocentesis may allow the aspiration of a few milliliters of blood, and this, along with rapid volume resuscitation to increase preload, can buy enough time to move to the operating room. However, in penetrating injury to the heart there is usually substantial clotting in the pericardium which may prevent aspiration. If there is no improvement, an urgent subxiphoid pericardial window, or thoracotomy is mandated.

It is better to perform a thoracotomy in the operating room, either through an anterolateral approach or a median sternotomy, with good light and assistance and the potential for autotransfusion and potential bypass than it is to attempt heroic emergency surgery in the resuscitation suite. However, if the patient is in extremis with a systolic blood pressure below 40 mmHg, despite volume resuscitation, proceed immediately with a left anterior thoracotomyin an attempt to relieve the tamponade and control the penetrating injury to the heart. If there is an obvious penetrating injury, the pericardium is opened to relieve any tamponade, and if there is injury to either the left or right ventricle, the wound can be digitally controlled. As a last resort, a Foley catheter can be introduced into the hole and the balloon distended to create tamponade. The end of the Foley catheter should be clamped. Great care should be taken to apply minimal traction on the Foley catheter, just enough to allow sealing. Excessive traction will pull the catheter out, and extend the wound by tearing the muscle.

Once the bleeding is controlled, the wound can be easily sutured with pledgetted sutures, or temporarily, with skin staples.

Hemorrhage from intercostal vessels, secondary to penetrating wounds (or multiple fractured ribs), frequently will stop without operative intervention. This is also true for most bleeding from the pulmonary system. However, careful monitoring is essential using an intra-thoracic drainage with an underwater seal, and if the bleeding persists, then thoracotomy will be required to control the bleeding. It is helpful to attempt to collect shed blood from the hemothorax into an autotransfusion collecting device so that the massive hemothorax can be immediately autotransfused to the patient, and if time and expertise permit, a double lumen endotracheal tube, is very helpful.

Transmediastinal Gunshot Injuries

These injuries carry a high mortality. The management decisions will depend on the hemodynamic stability of the patient, determining the tract of the bullet, and the potential for structures along that tract to have been damaged.

- In the stable patient, the best examination is a CT scan with contrast. This will help to determine both the track of the bullet and assist in deciding whether other investigations are required.
- An angiogram and contrast study of the esophagus are the minimum investigations required in the stable patient. However, modern multi-slice CT scanning with contrast is a suitable alternative.
- Echocardiography (including a trans-esophageal echocardiogram) may be helpful if the tract is near the heart.

Penetrating Injuries of the Abdomen

The delayed diagnosis and treatment of abdominal injuries is one of the most common causes of preventable death from blunt or penetrating trauma. The deaths usually result from continuing, uncontrolled hemorrhage. Not all penetrating injuries of the abdomen will require surgical intervention if the patient is hemodynamically stable.

It is important to appreciate the difference between surgical resuscitation and definitive treatment for abdominal trauma. Surgical resuscitation includes the technique of "damage control," and implies completion of only that surgery necessary to save life by stopping bleeding and preventing further contamination or injury.

Resuscitation

Resuscitation of patients with suspected abdominal injuries should always take place within the ATLS context. Attention is paid to adequate resuscitative measures, including adequate pain control. Adequate analgesia (titrated intravenously) will never mask abdominal symptoms, and is much more likely to make abdominal pathology easier to assess, with clearer physical signs and a co-operative patient.

Diagnosis

Blood is not initially an irritant, and therefore it may be difficult to assess the presence or quantity of blood present in the abdomen. Bowel sounds may remain present for several hours after abdominal injury, or may disappear following trivial trauma. This sign is therefore particularly unreliable.

Investigation and assessment of the abdomen can be based on three groups:

1. The patient with a normal abdomen
2. An equivocal group requiring further investigation
3. The patient with an obvious injury to the abdomen

In the presence of hypotension, virtually all penetrating injuries to the abdomen should be explored promptly. Diagnostic modalities depend on the nature of the injury.

- Physical examination
- Diagnostic peritoneal lavage (DPL)
- Ultrasound—focused abdominal sonography for trauma (FAST)
- Contrast enhanced computed tomography scan (CECT)
- Diagnostic laparoscopy

The Hemodynamically "Normal" Patient

There is ample time for a full evaluation of the patient, and a decision can be made regarding surgery or non-operative management.

The Hemodynamically "Stable" Patient

The stable patient, who is not hemodynamically normal, will benefit from investigations aimed at establishing answers to the following:

- Has the patient bled into the abdomen?
- Has the bleeding stopped?

Thus, serial investigations of a quantitative nature will allow the best assessment of these patients. CECT scan is currently the modality of choice, although FAST also may be helpful, but is dependent on the operator.

The Hemodynamically "Unstable" Patient

Efforts must be made to define the cavity where bleeding is taking place, e.g. chest, pelvis or abdominal cavity. Diagnostic modalities are limited out of necessity, since it may not be practical to move an unstable patient to CT scan, even if readily available. DPL remains one of the most common, sensitive, cheapest, and readily available modalities to assess the presence of blood in the abdomen. Importantly, DPL can be performed without moving the patient from the resuscitation area. FAST is similarly useful, but is more operator dependent (be cautious if the operator is inexperienced in trauma patient handling). It must be emphasized that a negative DPL carries much greater importance than a positive one, since it gives a very clear indication whether the bleeding is intraperitoneal in nature in the unstable patient. This situation lends itself to FAST examination, as hemodynamic instability caused by intraperitoneal hemorrhage is likely to be found at FAST examination, which may be somewhat quicker than DPL.

Management—Surgical Strategies

Selective conservatism in the management of stab wounds of the abdomen is well established. The patient is reassessed for peritonism by the same surgeon at a specified interval—usually 4 hourly. Failure to improve implies the need for surgical exploration. However, a degree of surgical experience is required, and the more inexperienced the surgeon is in the management of penetrating trauma, the more the policy should lean toward operative intervention. For gunshot injury, the standard treatment is laparotomy.

Surgery for abdominal injury can conveniently be divided into

- Patients who are hemodynamically stable with easily repairable injuries; should undergo appropriate definitive surgery.
- Patients who are hemodynamically unstable, or who have difficult injury complexes; should have a damage control procedure as their default initial surgery.

Damage Control (Abbreviated Laparotomy)

"Damage control," (also known as "staged laparotomy") is a surgical strategy that sacrifices the completeness of the immediate repair to allow time to address the combined physiological impact of trauma and surgery. Once the physiology has been optimized, then the definitive surgery can proceed.

Following most major torso trauma, there is gross physiological instability, characterized by hypothermia, coagulopathy and acidosis. The priorities are therefore to control any ongoing hemorrhage, and limit contamination (e.g. by bile or bowel content). Thereafter, resuscitation takes place in the intensive care setting. Once stability has been achieved, the patient is returned to the operating room. Although the principles are sound, extreme care has to be exercised in over-utilization of the concept so that secondary insults to the viscera are minimized. Furthermore, enough appropriate surgery has to be carried out initially, in order to minimize activation of the inflammatory cascade and the consequences of SIRS and organ dysfunction.

The concept is not new, and livers were packed as long as 90 years ago, but with a failure to understand the underlying rationale, the results were disastrous. The concept was reviewed and the technique of initial abortion of laparotomy, establishment of intra-abdominal pack tamponade, and then completion of the procedure (once coagulation has returned to an acceptable level) proved to be life-saving. The concept of staging applies both to routine and emergency procedures, and can work equally well in the chest, pelvis and neck as in the abdomen.

Stage 1: Patient selection

Indications for damage control are shown in Table 3.1. Irrespective of the setting, a coagulopathy is the most common reason for abortion of a planned procedure, or the curtailment of definitive surgery. It is important to abort the surgery before the coagulopathy becomes obvious, and possibly irreversible.

Stage 2: Operative hemorrhage and contamination control

The primary objectives are:

- Hemorrhage control
- Control of contamination
- Temporary closure of the abdomen

TABLE 3.1. Indications for damage control.

Anatomical	Inability to achieve hemostasis
	Complex abdominal injury, e.g. of liver and pancreas
	Combined vascular, solid and hollow organ injury, e.g. aortic or caval injury
	Inaccessible major venous injury, e.g. retrohepatic vena cava
	Demand for non operative control of other injuries, e.g. fractured pelvis
	Anticipated need for a time consuming procedure
Physiological	Temperature < 34°C
Decline of physiological reserve	pH < 7.2
	Serum lactate > 5 mmol/l (N < 2.5 mmol/l)
	PT > 16 s
	PTT > 60 s
	> 10 units blood transfused
	Systolic BP < 90 mmHg for more than 60 min
Environmental	Operating time greater than 60 min
	Inability to approximate the abdominal incision
	Desire to reassess the intra-abdominal contents (directed relook)

Stage 3: Physiological resuscitation in the ICU

Priorities in the ICU are:

- Restoration of body temperature
- Correction of the clotting profile
- Repletion of blood and its components
- Optimization of oxygenation of tissues
- Avoidance of abdominal compartment syndrome

Stage 4: Operative definitive surgery

The patient is returned to the operating theater as soon as Stage 3 is achieved, which should take place within 48 h. The timing is determined by:

- The indication for damage control in the first place
- The injury pattern
- The physiological response

Stage 5: Abdominal wall reconstruction

Once the patient has received definitive surgery, and no further operations are contemplated, then the abdominal wall can be closed.

Irrespective of the nature of both the initial and definitive surgeries which takes place, adjuncts such as adequate early nutrition (preferably enteral) optimized lung ventilation, tissue perfusion, and due attention to the immunosuppression associated with trauma patients will ensure the best possible outcome.

Selected Readings

Ellis BW, Paterson-Brown S (eds) (2000) Hamilton Bailey's emergency surgery, 13th edn. Arnold, London

Garden OJ, Paterson Brown S (ed) Abdominal Trauma (2005) Core Topics in General and Emergency Surgery: A companion to specialist surgical practice: 3rd edn. W.B. Saunders, London

Moore EE, Feliciano DV, Mattox LK (eds) (2004) Trauma, 5th edn. McGraw Hill, New York

Practice Management Guidelines. Eastern Association for the Surgery of Trauma www.east.org (accessed 2006)

Russell RCG, Williams NN, Bulstrode CJK (eds) (2004) Bailey and Love's short practice of surgery, 24th edn. Arnold, London

4

Vascular Trauma: Life-threatening Thoracoabdominal Injuries and Limb-threatening Extremity Injuries

C. Clay Cothren and Ernest E. Moore

Pearls and Pitfalls

- Prompt diagnosis based on injury mechanism and systematic evaluation in the emergency department for the 6 Ps:
  - Pallor
  - Paresthesia
  - Pulselessness
  - Paralysis
  - Pain
  - Poikilothermic

- Secure initial control of hemorrhage with digital compression
- Obtain early proximal and distal vascular control
- Arterial shunt quickly if delayed presentation
- Intraoperative angiography for diagnosis and evaluation of repair
- Presumptive fasciotomy
- Know regional nerve anatomy

Vascular injury can produce rapid exsanguination and threaten extremities or it may be a clinically silent time bomb with potentially disastrous consequences. Thus, a high index of suspicion, prompt diagnosis, and appropriate intervention

K.I. Bland et al. (eds.), *Trauma Surgery*,
DOI 10.1007/978-1-84996-375-6_4,
© Springer-Verlag London Limited 2011

are crucial to minimize associated morbidity and mortality. Although specific mechanisms of trauma should alert the practicing surgeon to unique injury patterns, identifying and managing the particular zone of injury is the most applicable information for the reader.

Thoracic Vascular Trauma

Almost a quarter of trauma-related deaths are due to thoracic injuries, and the vast majority of these injuries occur after penetrating mechanisms. Patients with penetrating wounds of the great vessels often present with massive hemorrhage or cardiac tamponade, while blunt injuries may be more subtle in their presentation. Hemodynamic instability and clinically significant chest tube output (>1,500 ml initial)represent indications for immediate thoracotomy. Mechanism of injury, patient symptoms, and clinical signs dictate ancillary imaging to evaluate for occult thoracic vascular injury.

Innominate Artery

Blunt innominate artery injury typically follows rapid deceleration mechanisms such as head-on motor vehicle collisions. The initial chest film may reveal a right-sided mediastinal hematoma (Fig. 4.1.) rather than the classic left-sided hematoma associated with descending thoracic aortic (DTA) injuries. The anatomy of the aortic arch and precise location and type of injury, either pseudoaneurysm or arterial avulsion, is clarified with angiography. The ideal operative approach is through a median sternotomy with or without a cervical extension. After thoracic entry and prior to exploration of the hematoma, an 8 mm polytetrafluoroethylene (PTFE) graft should be placed between the proximal aorta and the distal, transected innominate artery. Cardiac bypass and anticoagulation can be avoided with the use of a side-biting Satinsky clamp on the aortic arch during the proximal anastomosis. The innominate vein may be divided to acquire adequate visualization, or the tube

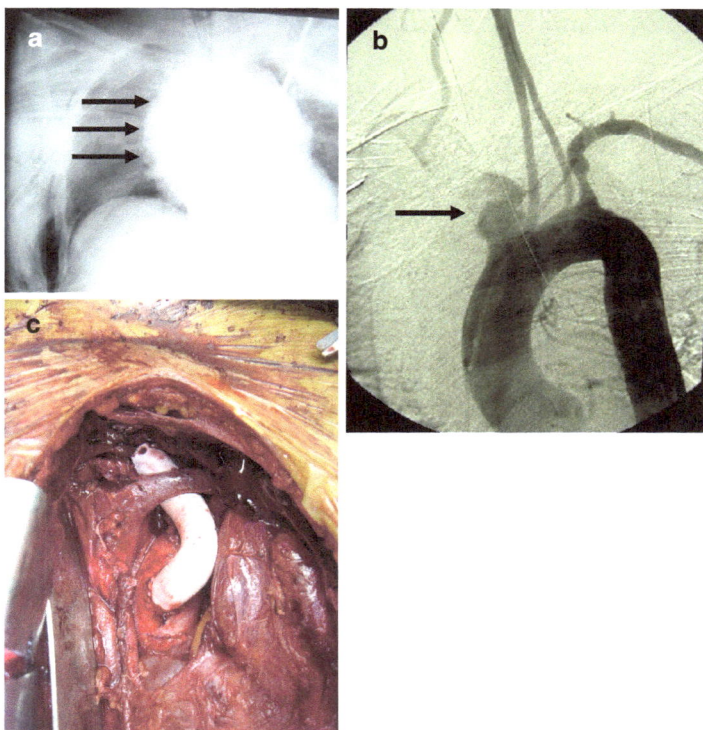

FIGURE 4.1. Post-injury imaging of the innominate artery reveals a right-sided mediastinal hematoma (**a**) and either a pseudoaneurysm or free extravasation at the innominate takeoff (**b**). Polytetra-fluoroethylene (PTFE) "jump-graft" is placed between the proximal aorta and the distal, transected innominate artery, passing underneath the innominate vein (**c**).

graft can be passed underneath it. After graft interposition, the innominate injury is explored, controlled, and oversewn flush with the aortic arch. In patients sustaining penetrating injuries with hemodynamic instability or clinically significant chest-tube output, control of hemorrhage becomes the primary focus and maybe obtained initially with digital control, followed by a side-biting Satinsky clamp beneath the area of injury, and then standard "jump-graft" off the proximal aorta.

Subclavian and Axillary Artery

Common patterns of injury to the subclavian artery are transection after a gunshot or stab wound to the upper chest, arterial thrombosis due to a blunt stretch injury, or direct injury due to a clavicular fracture. Only 21% of patients have an upper extremity pulse differential; therefore, patients considered high-risk due to mechanism or proximity should be evaluated with high-resolution computed tomography angiography (CTA) (Fig. 4.2). As associated injuries of the brachial plexus are common, a thorough neurologic examination of the extremity is mandated prior to operative intervention.

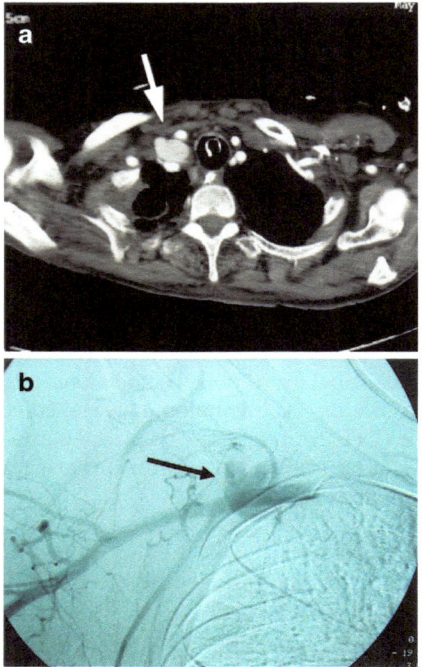

FIGURE 4.2. Imaging of subclavian artery wounds show a suspicious hematoma in proximity to the vessels (**a**) or overt evidence of injury on angiography (**b**).

Adequate exposure of the proximal subclavian artery is best obtained via a median sternotomy on the right and a left anterior thoracotomy with upper sternal extension on the left. Repair of the distal subclavian artery is performed in two steps. To prevent exsanguination when approaching the injury, proximal arterial control is acquired with a 6 cm supra-clavicular incision, encircling the subclavian artery with a vessel loop, while avoiding the phrenic nerve. Rapid exposure with a large hematoma may require proximal clavicular transection or resection. Adequate exposure of the injury is then obtained through an infraclavicular incision, extending out onto the upper arm as needed, with separation of the fibers of the pectoralis major muscle. Indiscriminate ligation or clamping for bleeding without identification of the culprit vessel could result in inadvertent injury to the intertwined cords of the brachial plexus. Either a reversed saphenous vein graft or 6 mm PTFE graft is appropriate for repair.

Descending Thoracic Aorta

Approximately 10% of deaths after motor vehicle crashes (MVCs) are due to blunt tears in the DTA. The most common mechanisms are high-speed, head-on collisions or side impacts, although DTA injuries may be seen with autopedestrians' struck, fall, or crush injuries. Blunt injuries are located typically in the proximal descending aorta, just beyond the subclavian artery at the ligamentum arteriosum. Due to shear forces, there is typically partial transection of the aorta with contain-ment by the pleural envelope preventing exsanguination. Occasionally complete transection or intimal dissection of the aorta with false lumen extension occurs. Suggestive findings on chest radiograph include loss of the aortic knob, mediastinal widening, apical capping, blurring of the aortopulmonary window, and deviation of trachea (Fig. 4.3). Computed tomography (CT) and digital reconstructions are now the standard for definitive diagnosis. Patients with a concerning mechanism of injury should be started on intravenous beta-blockade in the emergency department prior to diagnostic

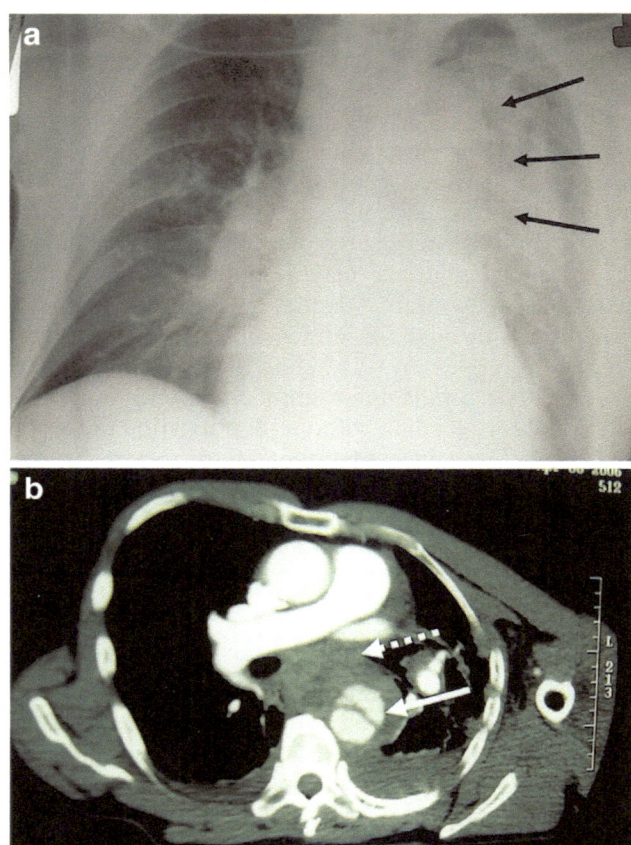

FIGURE 4.3. Descending thoracic aortic (DTA) tears result in a widened mediastinum (**a**) on chest radiograph; computed tomography (CT) of the chest (**b**) documents partial aortic transection with intimal flap (solid arrow) and associated periaortic hematoma (dashed line).

imaging to decrease shear stress on the aortic wall; a short-acting agent, e.g., esmolol, is the drug of choice, with the goal of decreasing systemic blood pressure to ≤ 100 mmHg and heart rate to < 100/min.

Current options for acute DTA tears include nonoperative management for minor injuries and endovascular stenting in patients with complex multisystem trauma, but operative repair remains the current standard. After double-lumen endotracheal intubation, operative access is acquired through a left posterolateral thoracotomy. The patient's hips are pivoted toward a supine 45° angle to provide access to the left femoral vessels for partial left heart bypass or femoral venoarterial bypass. Although primary repair with or without a graft patch is occasionally feasible, the majority of injuries require inter-position grafting. Key pitfalls to be avoided during operation include the phrenic and vagus nerves during subclavian dissection and a left-sided recurrent laryngeal nerve (if present) during aortic repair. Centrifugal pumps for bypass do not require full systemic anticoagulation, but low-dose heparin (100u/kg) is usually administered unless there are substantive intracranial or spinal injuries or major solid organ injuries. Several clinical scenarios may modify the operative approach to the torn DTA. In the event of ongoing hemorrhage from concomitant abdominal trauma, emergent laparotomy is done prior to aortic repair, and unrelenting bleeding from pelvic fractures would similarly assume precedence. In patients with life-threatening intracranial bleeding or extensive right pulmonary contusion precluding left lung compression, the decision making becomes complicated. Nonoperative management with blood pressure control has proven safe and effective for some DTA tears, but head injury will not frequently permit hypotension. In these patients, endovascular stenting is probably the optimal management. In fact, endovascular repair may soon become the preferred treatment of DTA lesions.

Abdominal Vascular Trauma

A wide range of patient symptoms are encountered with intra-abdominal injuries, but most manifest some evidence of acute blood loss. With penetrating wounds to the abdomen, identification of the source of hemorrhage is usually accomplished at the time of emergent laparotomy. Initial vascular control should be accomplished with digital compression, with vascular clamps placed thereafter proximally and distally when feasible. Alternatively, if the vascular injury is contained, wide exposure and proximal/distal control should be gained before entering the hematoma. Associated open-bowel injuries, common with penetrating wounds, should be addressed by rapid stapling to minimize ongoing contamination. It is important to recognize that synthetic graft infections in the abdomen, despite associated gastrointestinal contamination, are rare.

Abdominal Aorta

Patients who survive to reach the operating room (OR) with a penetrating aortic wound frequently have a contained hematoma or free hemorrhage into the abdomen. For supra-renal aortic injuries, a left medial visceral rotation is essential for adequate exposure; if the injury is supraceliac, transecting the left crus of the diaphragm or performing left thoracotomy may be necessary. Due to lack of mobility of the abdominal aorta, few injuries are amenable to primary repair; small lateral perforations may be controlled with 4–0 prolene suture or a PTFE patch. But end-to-end interposition grafting with a PTFE tube graft is the most common repair. In contrast, blunt injuries are typically intimal tears of the infrarenal aorta and are exposed readily via a direct approach. To avoid future vascular-enteric fistulas, the vascular suture lines should be covered with mesentery or omentum.

Superior Mesenteric Artery and Vein

Penetrating wounds to the superior mesenteric artery (SMA) are encountered typically when exploring the abdomen for a gunshot wound, with "black bowel" and associated suprames-ocolic hematoma being pathognomonic (Fig. 4.4). Blunt avulsion of the SMA is rare but should be queried in patients with a seatbelt-sign who have mid-epigastric pain or tenderness and associated hypotension. Operative approach, regardless of the etiology of injury, is based on the level of SMA injury.

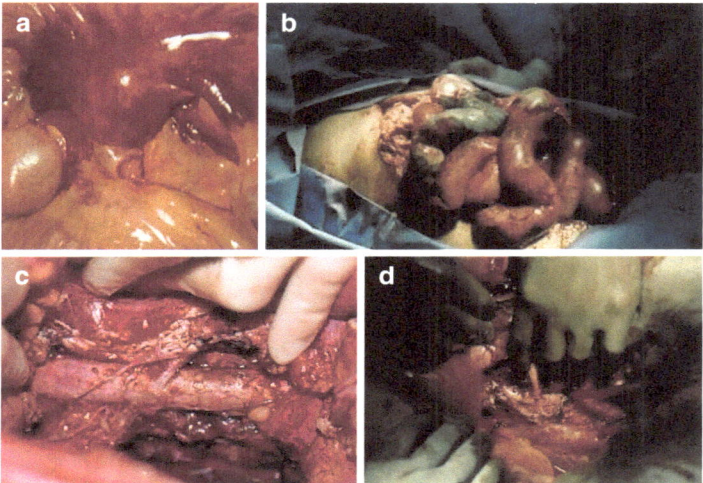

FIGURE 4.4. A supramesocolic hematoma (**a**) with associated "black bowel" (**b**) is pathognomonic for wounds to the superior mesenteric artery (SMA). Operative approach of Fullen zone I SMA injuries are exposed by a left medial visceral rotation, exposing the length of the aorta (**c**). Definitive repair is with a polytetrafluoroethylene (PTFE) graft from the aorta to the SMA past the point of injury (**d**).

Fullen zone I injuries of the SMA, posterior to the pancreas, can be exposed by a left medial visceral rotation leaving the left kidney in situ. Fullen zone II SMA injuries, from the pancreatic edge to the middle colic branch, are approached via the lesser sac along the inferior edge of the pancreas at the base of the transverse mesocolon; the pancreatic body may be divided to gain proximal vascular access. More distal SMA injuries, Fullen zone III/IV, are approached directly and repaired within the mesentery.

For injuries of the SMA, temporary damage control with a Pruitt shunt can prevent bowel ischemia and edema; additionally, temporary shunting allows control of visceral contamination prior to placement of a PTFE graft. For definitive repair, end-to-end interposition with a reversed saphenous vein graft from the proximal SMA to the SMA past the point of injury can be done if there is no associated pancreatic injury. Alternatively, if the patient has an associated pancreatic injury, the graft should be tunneled from the distal aorta beneath the duodenum to the SMA. For proximal SMV injuries, digital compression for control of hemorrhage is followed by attempted venorrhaphy; ligation is an option in a life-threatening situation, but resultant bowel edema requires aggressive fluid resuscitation. Temporary abdominal closure and a second-look operation to evaluate bowel viability should be done.

Portal Triad

Penetrating wounds to the structures of the portal triad are the most common mechanism of injury, but blunt avulsions can occur. In general, the celiac axis to the level of common hepatic artery at the gastroduodenal arterial branch maybe ligated due to extensive collaterals, but the proper hepatic artery should be repaired. The right or left hepatic artery, or in urgent situations the portal vein, may be ligated selectively, but associated ischemia of the liver parenchyma may necessitate delayed resection. If the right hepatic artery is ligated, cholecystectomy should also be performed. To gain access to the portal structures, control should first be gained with a Pringle maneuver prior to entering a hematoma; after defining the level of injury, vascular clamps facilitate exposure and should be used for proximal and distal control. Blindly suturing mon bile duct. If the vascular injury is a stab wound with clean transection of the vessels, primary end-to-end repair is done. If the injury is destructive, temporary shunting should be performed followed by interposition-reversed saphenous vein graft. Blunt avulsions of the portal structures are particularly problematic if located at the hepatic plate, flush with the liver; control of hemorrhage at the liver can be attempted with directed packing or use of Fogarty catheters. If the avulsion is more proximal-flush with the pancreatic body border or if retropancreatic-the pancreas must be transected to gain access for control of the hemorrhage and repair.

Renovascular

Penetrating wounds to the renal pedicle are frequently destructive, and the initial priority is to control bleeding from the aorta and vena cava with Satinsky vascular clamps. In patients with multiple intra-abdominal injuries, nephrectomy is warranted. But the kidney should not be discarded until a normal functioning contralateral kidney is confirmed. The approach to blunt renal artery occlusion is controversial; renal salvage is rare if the warm ischemia time exceeds 5 h. Furthermore, most of these lesions are in the juxtaaortic renal artery and can be technically quite challenging.

Vascular Trauma of the Extremity

Often the extremities are placed at the bottom of the "to-do" list in patients with life-threatening multisystem trauma, only to find an ischemic limb hours later. Therefore, a high index of suspicion is warranted in patients with extremity fracture/dislocations; careful peripheral vascular examination, including Doppler pressure measurements comparing extremities, and associated neurologic examination is mandatory prior to transport to the OR or for ancillary imaging. Blunt trauma results in a stretch injury and subsequent occlusion of the artery at the level of the associated fracture or joint dislocation. Penetrating wounds can produce either vessel transection ora pseudoaneurysm. Motor/sensory defects may be the first sign of arterial injury due to ischemia, rather than an absent pulse. Additionally, imaging patients with soft signs or those with penetrating injuries in proximity to major vascular structures are important to avoid delays. Angiography, to discern between vessel spasm and overt injury, can be performed in the angiography suite or in the OR. "On-table" angiography in the OR facilitates rapid intervention, and is warranted in patients with evidence of ischemia on arrival in the emergency department. The notable exception is the patient with multiple fracture sites. Arterial access for "on-table" lower extremity angiography can be obtained percutaneously at the femoral vessels with a standard arterial catheter, via femoral vessel exposure and direct cannulation, or with exposure of the superficial femoral artery just above the medial knee. Once the vessel is repaired and restoration of arterial flow documented, completion angiography should be done in the OR if there is no palpable distal pulse.

Vasoparalysis with verapamil, nitroglycerine, and papaverin may be employed. Fasciotomy, most often employed in the lower extremity, should be considered for all ischemic periods greater than 6 h or combined injury of named arteries and accompanying veins. Nonoperative management for small intimal flaps is appropriate, but repeated clinical follow-up is mandatory.

Brachial Artery

Brachial artery injuries are usually due to penetrating mechanisms (stab wounds, gunshot wounds, plate glass window laceration), and paramedics typically report substantial blood loss at the scene or pulsatile bleeding from the open wound. Blunt injuries with intimal dissections and secondary thrombosis may occur in patients with supracondylar fractures of the humerus. Although exploration is indicated in the majority of penetrating injuries, angiography may be helpful to diagnose blunt occlusions (Fig. 4.5). Operative approach for a brachial artery injury is via a medial, upper extremity longitudinal incision; proximal control may be obtained at the axillary artery, and an S-shaped extension through the antecubital fossa provides access to the distal brachial artery. The segment of injured vessel is excised, and an end-to-end interposition using reverse saphenous vein is the procedure of choice. Upper extremity fasciotomy is required only rarely, unless the patient manifests preoperative neurologic changes, diminished pulse on revascularization, or extended time frame to operative intervention. Temporary shunting with a Pruitt-Inahara shunt may be useful for patient transport to an experienced facility.

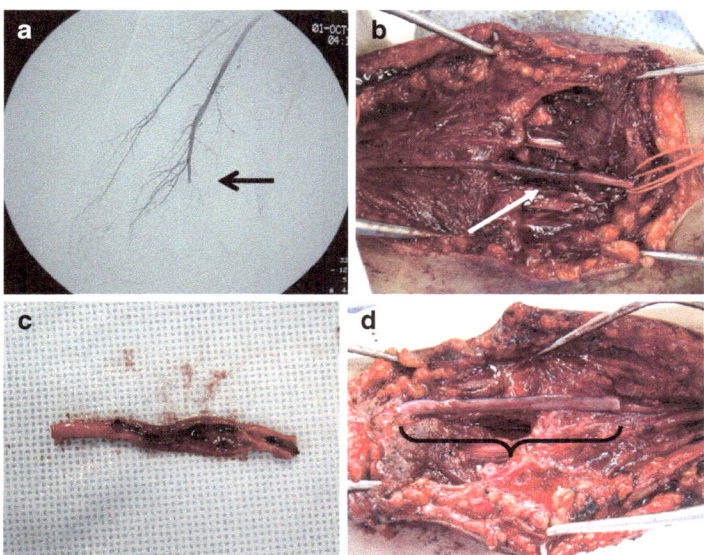

FIGURE 4.5. Angiography confirms blunt brachial artery occlusion (**a**). On exploration via a medial upper extremity longitudinal incision, external bruising at the site of occlusion is evident (**b**). The injured vessel segment, with associated dissection and thrombosis, is excised (**c**) and an end-to-end interposition reversed saphenous vein graft is performed (**d**).

External Iliac Artery

Transpelvic gunshot wounds or blunt injuries with associated pelvic fractures are the most common scenarios in patients with iliac artery injuries. Clinical examination and pulse measurements usually suggest the underlying injury, with confirmatory pelvic angiography employed occasionally (Fig. 4.6). Operative exposure via a transabdominal approach affords access to the level of the inguinal ligament; a counter-incision in the groin may be used to acquire more distal access. A Javid shunt can be used for damage control, with temporary shunting of the vessel. Definitive interposition

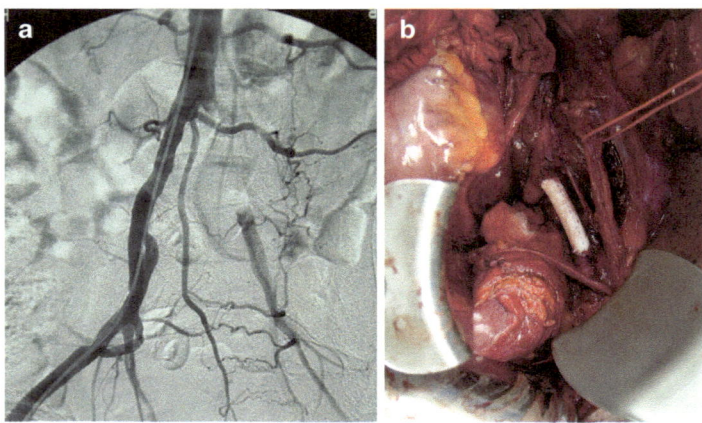

FIGURE 4.6. Pelvic angiography reveals acute thrombosis of the left iliac artery (**a**) which is repaired with interposition tube grafting via a transabdominal approach (**b**).

tube grafting with excision of the injured segment is appropriate. Careful monitoring for distal embolic events and reperfusion injury necessitating fasciotomy is imperative.

Superficial Femoral Artery

Although penetrating injury may result in transection with obvious signs of hemorrhage, a more insidious presentation of injury to the superficial femoral artery is seen in patients with a distal femur fracture after blunt trauma (Fig. 4.7). The superficial femoral artery may either have intimal injury with thrombosis or complete blunt transection. Therefore, it is imperative to always ascertain ankle–ankle (A–A) indices after reduction of femur fractures in the trauma bay. If the A–A index is <0.9, angiography is indicated to evaluate for injury versus vessel spasm. Clearly, if the patient has a threatened foot, on-table angiography in the OR or operative exploration at fracture site should be performed. Typically, external fixation of the femur is performed followed by end-to-end reversed

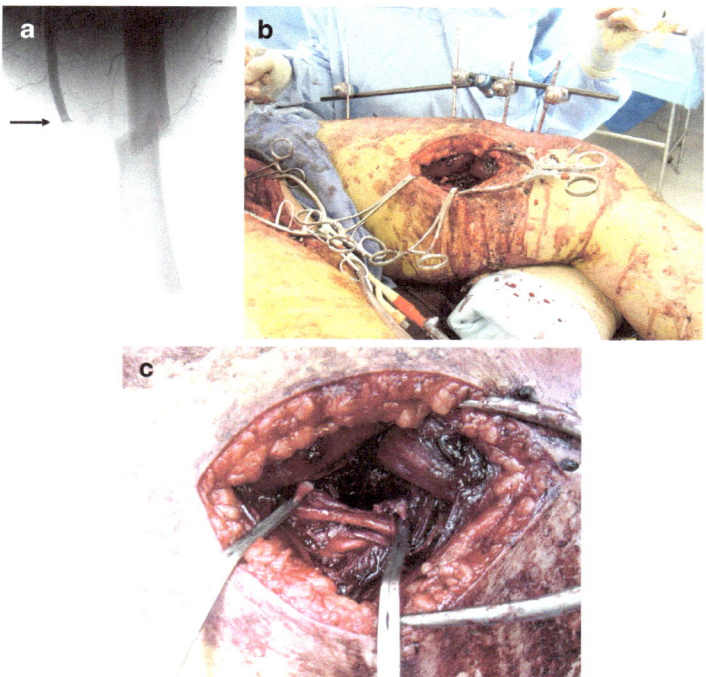

FIGURE 4.7. Thrombosis of the superficial femoral artery occurs at the level of the distal femur fracture (**a**). After external fixation of the femur, a medial approach is used for exposure (**b**) and excision of the injured arterial segment (**c**).

saphenous vein graft of the injured segment of the superficial femoral artery. Temporary shunting of the superficial femoral artery maybe performed during orthopedic manipulation, particularly if there is a delay in recognition. Close monitoring for calf compartment syndrome is mandatory.

Popliteal Artery

Popliteal artery injuries are common after knee dislocations or supracondylar femur fractures in children (which clinically mimic knee dislocations). After relocation and maintaining alignment of the knee, clinical and pulse examination is performed. If the A–A index is <0.9, or if there are diminished pulses in the foot, angiography should be performed; however, clear ischemic compromise mandates immediate operative exploration. Preferred access to the popliteal space for an acute injury is the medial approach with one incision which allows detaching of the semitendinosus, semimembranosus, and gracilis tendons (Fig. 4.8). Other options include a straight posterior approach with an

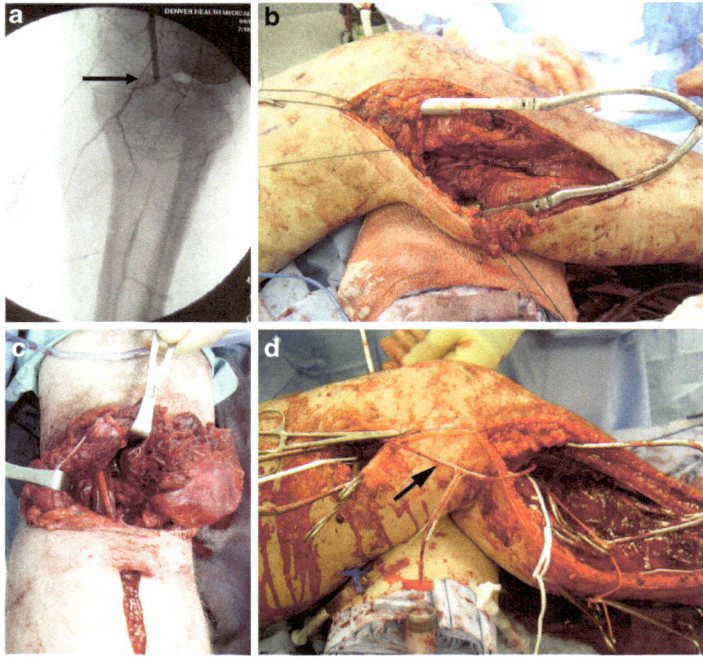

FIGURE 4.8. After reduction of a posterior knee dislocation, angiography should be performed to evaluate for a popliteal artery injury if the A–A index is <0.9 (**a**). Access to the popliteal vessel is either the medial approach (**b**) or the straight posterior approach with an S-shaped incision (**c**). Rapid temporary shunting in compromised extremities can be performed with a medial approach with two incisions (**d**).

S-shaped incision and a medial approach with two incisions. If the patient has an associated popliteal vein injury, this vein should be repaired first with a PTFE interposition graft while the artery is shunted. For an isolated popliteal artery injury, a reversed saphenous vein graft is performed either with an end-to-end or end-to-side proximal anastomosis and an end-to-end distal anastomosis. Compartment syndrome is common, and presumptive four-compartment fasciotomies are warranted in the majority of patients with combined arterial/venous injury.

Post-Injury Considerations

Although outcome is related to the technical success of the operation, in general the main cause of patient morbidity and mortality is associated soft tissue and nerve injury. Therefore, optimizing the patient's hemodynamic status, maintaining euthermia, and correcting coagulopathy are critical points of resuscitation. Prosthetic graft infections are rare complications, but preventing bacteremia is clearly imperative; administration of perioperative antibiotics and treatment of secondary infections are also indicated. Long-term arterial graft complications, such as stenosis or pseudoaneurysms, are uncommon, and routine graft surveillance is performed rarely. Consequently, long-term antiplatelet agents or antithrombotics are not routine.

Selected Readings

Carroll PR, McAninch JW, Klosterman P, Greenblatt M (1984) Renovascular trauma: risk assessment, surgical management, and outcome. J Trauma 30:547

Courcy PA, Brotman S, Oster-Grantie ML, et al. (1984) Superior mesenteric artery and vein injuries from blunt abdominal trauma. J Trauma 24:843

Dajee H, Richardson IW, Iype MO (1979) Seatbelt aorta: acute dissection and thrombosis of the abdominal aorta. Surgery 85:263

Feliciano DV (1998) Approach to major abdominal vascular injury. J Vasc Surg 7:730

Fullen WD, Hunt J, Altermeier WA (1972) The clinical spectrum of penetrating injury to the superior mesenteric arterial circulation. J Trauma 12:656

Johnston RH, Wall MJ, Mattox KL (1993) Innominate artery trauma: a thirty-year experience. J Vasc Surg 17:134

Kavic SM, Atweb N, Ivy ME, et al. (2001) Celiac axis ligation after gunshot wound to the abdomen: case report and review of the literature. J Trauma 50:738

Marin ML, Veith FJ, Panetta TF, et al. (1994) Transluminally placed endovascular stented graft repair for trauma. JVasc Surg 20:466

Petersen SF, Sheldon GF, Lim RC (1979) Management of portal vein injuries. J Trauma 19:616

Reber PU, Patel AG, Sapio NLD, et al. (1999) Selective us of temporary intravascular shunts in coincident vascular and orthopedic upper and lower limb trauma. J Trauma 47:72

5
Thermal Injury

Nora F. Nugent and David N. Herndon

Pearls and Pitfalls

- Burn wounds can be categorized into superficial, partial -thickness, and full-thickness injuries to skin, depending on depth of injury to the epidermis and dermis.
- The severity of a burn is determined largely by the depth of injury and the extent or percentage of total body surface area involved.
- Areas such as the face, hands, feet, and perineum have special considerations in terms of functional and cosmetic outcomes.
- When assessing a large burn, a primary survey starting with airway, breathing, and circulation (ABC) must be done as in any trauma patient, with each problem encountered treated adequately.
- Early and adequate fluid resuscitation is vital and improves outcome in large burns.
- Burn patients may have sustained other injuries during their thermal injury. Do not forget to fully assess the patient.
- In circumferential, full thickness burns of the thorax and extremities, escharotomies may be necessary to allow adequate ventilation and circulation.
- In children and the elderly or incapacitated, consider non-accidental injury for suspicious injuries.
- Superficial and partial-thickness wounds may be treated with topical ointments and dressings.

K.I. Bland et al. (eds.), *Trauma Surgery*,
DOI 10.1007/978-1-84996-375-6_5,
© Springer-Verlag London Limited 2011

• Deep dermal and full-thickness burns need surgical debridement and skin grafting. The wound may be covered temporarily with allo- or xenograft.

Basic Science

The pathophysiology of a thermal injury can be divided into that which occurs at a local level at the area of injury and the systemic response that occurs with a larger injury. Within the burn wound, three zones of injury have been described. An innermost zone of coagulation denotes an area of irreversible tissue loss, as a result of protein coagulation and denaturation. Surrounding this area is the zone of stasis, a region of potentially salvageable tissue. Damage has occurred, and there is decreased tissue perfusion. Resuscitation can prevent damage in this zone from becoming irreversible, however, conversely, inadequate resuscitation, infection, or excessive edema formation can convert possibly viable tissue to nonviable tissue. Prolonged decreased perfusion can lead to increased local tissue ischemia. Loss of tissue here can result in the burn wound deepening and widening. The outermost zone is the zone of hyperemia, in which as the name suggests, there is increased tissue perfusion, vasodilatation, and microvascular permeability. Inflammation and edema formation can take place here. This area of tissue recovers usually from injury.

After a burn reaches approximately 30% of the total body surface area, the effect of cytokine and inflammatory mediator release at the site of injury begins to have a systemic effect. Massive tissue edema can occur in burned tissue and also in unburned areas of soft tissue, intestine, lung, and muscle. The increased pressure in the tissue from the accumulated fluid can lead to decreased perfusion and subsequent ischemia, particularly in circumferential limb burns, especially full-thickness injuries, as deeper tissues (muscle, nerve) may become ischemic and require surgical release. This phenomenon occurs as a consequence of factors affecting control of transcapillary fluid shifts and fluid accumulation in the interstitium. Intravascular volume depletion transpires rapidly unless fluid resuscitation is adequate, although over-resuscitation can accentuate the edema formation. The rate of edema formation can be very rapid. Some of the factors involved include a marked increase in the rate of fluid and protein crossing into the interstitium, a marked increase in capillary permeability, inability to maintain a plasma-to-interstitial oncotic gradient, a decrease in interstitial pressure secondary to the release of osmotically active particles causing a vacuum effect pulling fluid in from plasma, and early disruption of the integrity of the interstitial space with disorder of collagen and hyaluronic acid structures and progressive increase in interstitial space compliance.

Myocardial contractility is decreased, possibly due to release of tumor necrosis factor a. The basal metabolic rate of the body increases to up to three times its original rate and leads to a catabolic state with loss of lean muscle mass. Downregulation of the body's immune response occurs, affecting both cell-mediated and humeral pathways. Bacterial translocation can arise from an impaired gastrointestinal mucosal barrier.

Carbon monoxide poisoning may also be present impairing oxygenation. Lung injury can occur as part of an inhalation injury or as a systemic reaction to the burn injury. Direct thermal injury from superheated gas and liquids can damage the upper airway. Airway obstruction and edema results from this topical epithelial injury and from the diffuse capillary leak associated with a cutaneous burn. Bronchospasm may be triggered by irritating chemicals inhaled, and small airway obstruction can result from sloughed epithelium, debris, and accumulated secretions, because the usual clearing ciliary mechanism is impaired. Alveolar collapse and atelectasis then occur as can pulmonary edema. This series of events leads to a high risk of tracheobronchitis and pneumonia, the end stage of which can be respiratory failure.

Clinical Presentation

The clinical presentation of thermal injury can vary depending on the causal agent and the depth and extent of the injury. An inhalation injury may accompany the cutaneous injury.

TABLE 5.1. Characteristics of different depths of thermal injury.

Depth of burn	Skin appearance	Blisters	Capillary refill	Sensation
Superficial	Red	No	Rapid	Painful
Superficial partial thickness	Pink, moist	Yes	Present	Painful
Deep partial thickness	Pink, blotchy, dry	Sometimes	Slow	Reduced
Full thickness	White or black, dry	No	Absent	Absent

The appearance of the burned area varies according to the depth of the burn (Table 5.1).

First degree or superficial thermal injury involves only the epidermis. First degree burns present as pain and erythema of the skin, and generally heal within a week without scarring. Second degree or partial-thickness injury, which involves damage to both the epidermis and to a variable degree the underlying dermis, can be divided into superficial and deep categories. In superficial partial-thickness burns, the epidermis and no deeper than the upper third of the dermis is injured. Typically, there is blistering, and the wound is very painful, moist, and pink and blanches readily on pressure. Serous fluid usually oozes from the wound (Figs. 5.1 and 5.2). Deep partial-thickness burns incur destruction of the epidermis and most of the dermis. These burns have a pink to white appearance and are not as painful as their more superficial counterparts because nerve endings have been injured. Capillary refill is reduced and may be very difficult to see.

Full-thickness or third degree injury is where the epidermis and the entire dermis are burned. The wound has a white, waxy appearance or a charred leathery eschar (Fig. 5.3), is not painful because the nerve endings have been destroyed, and does not blanch on pressure. Coagulated vessels may be visible. Sometimes, it is very difficult to distinguish deep partial-thickness injury from third degree. Subdermal or fourth degree wounds occur when the injury has penetrated into the subcutaneous tissue and may involve muscle, tendon, or bone.

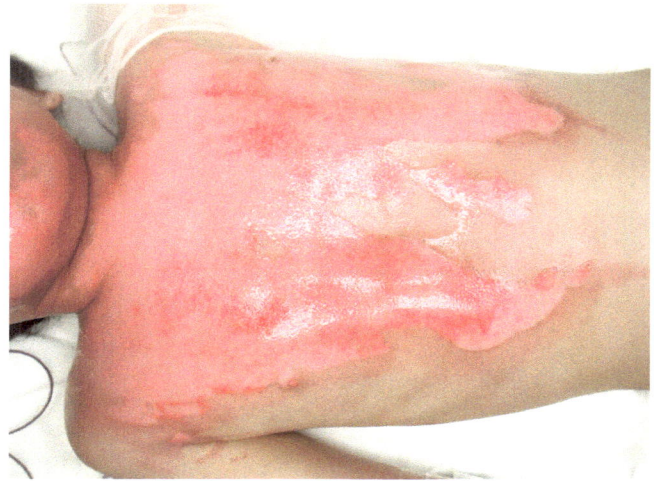

FIGURE 5.1. Superficial burn to anterior chest from a scald injury.

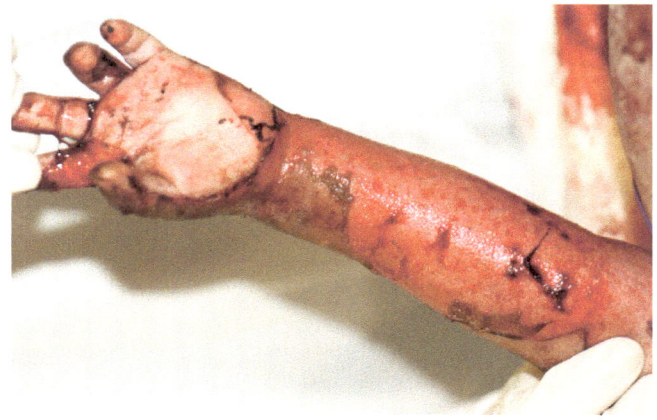

FIGURE 5.2. Partial-thickness burn to forearm and hand.

The mechanism of injury affects the clinical presentation and subsequent management. Flame injuries tend to produce full-or partial-thickness injuries. These burns may result from house fires or accidents with flammable substances such as

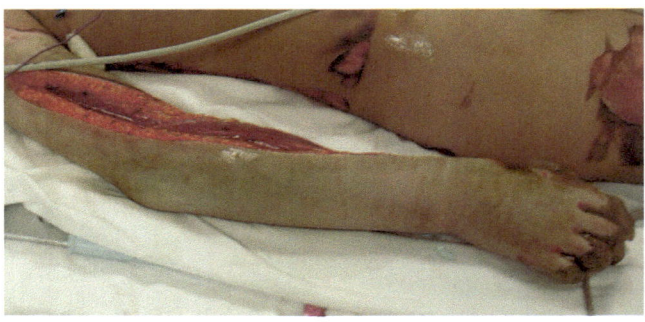

FIGURE 5.3. Full-thickness burn to upper extremity. Escharotomies and fasciotomies have been performed.

gasoline. Scald injuries are common in children and tend to produce superficial and partial thickness injuries. Contact burns, which result from prolonged contact with a hot surface or contact with an extremely hot surface, tend to be deep dermal or full-thickness. These burns are seen usually in children or those who cannot remove themselves quickly from the source, such as the elderly, epileptics during a seizure, the disabled, or those under intoxication.

Electrical injuries vary in severity depending on the voltage of the power source. Low voltages, e.g. domestic electricity, usually cause small, deep contact entry and exit site burns. An alternating current crossing the myocardium has the potential to trigger cardiac arrhythmias. High voltages cause much more extensive tissue destruction. As well as entry and exit point burns, extensive muscle necrosis and nerve damage can occur along the path of the current. Limb loss may occur. Rhabdomyolysis from muscle damage and renal failure can also result from the injury. If the victim does not actually make contact with the power source, but is very close by, a flash injury can occur from an arc of current. The heat of the flash can cause superficial burns and can set clothing on fire resulting in deeper burns.

Chemical injuries occur as a result of contact with acids or alkalis, either in the workplace or the home. These burns tend to be deep and can penetrate tissue progressively if the chemical persists on the skin and continues to injure the tissue. Acid burns are painful and cause a coagulative necrosis and protein denaturation. Of note, hydrofluoric acid (used in glass etching) reacts with the body's calcium and can rapidly cause fatal hypocalcemia. Alkali burns induce a liquefactive necrosis and can penetrate deeper into tissues than acid. The onset of pain may be delayed, allowing the chemical longer contact with the skin before treatment is initiated.

Substantive inhalation injury usually presents with signs and symptoms of upper airway distress, such as stridor and dysphonia, from the resultant mucosal edema. Symptoms usually occur after some time has passed because it takes time for the edema to accumulate. Indications that an airway injury may have occurred include face and neck burns, singed nasal and facial hairs, and the presence of carbonaceous material in the mouth and upper airway. Symptoms of carbon monoxide poisoning may range from disorientation to obtundation and coma, depending on the extent of poisoning.

Diagnosis

Diagnosis of a thermal injury is based largely on history and physical examination. A thorough assessment and evaluation of the patient is essential. For a large burn, it may be necessary to begin emergency management while evaluating the patient concurrently.

In the history, the following information should be asked: the cause of the thermal injury, the time at which it occurred, whether the victim was in an enclosed space, and the duration of contact with the injuring agent. Any other injuries sustained at the time should be inquired about and sought after, because the patient may have other injuries sustained due to the nature of the injury, such as an explosion, or while trying to jump to escape from a burning house. Tetanus status should be established, and any first aid or other medical attention received at the scene enquired about. Allergies, medications, and pre-existing medical conditions also need to be known.

The severity of a burn injury is determined largely by the depth and extent of the burn injury. Notable exceptions to this include some chemical burns, such as hydrofluoric acid, and electrical injuries. The depth of injury is determined by the physical appearance of the cutaneous injury, and as discussed earlier can be classified into superficial, partial-thickness, and full-thickness injuries. This assessment is generally a clinical one, but techniques such as biopsies, laser Doppler studies, and ultrasonography, have been used in certain occasions to determine depth of injury.

The extent of burn injury is determined by calculating the percentage total body surface area (% TBSA) involved. Erythema or first-degree thermal injury is not included in this calculation. Several methods have been used to determine % TBSA involvement. The "rule of nines" can be used for a quick calculation, where each upper limb is 9%, each lower limb 18% etc. This general rule, however, does not take into account the different proportions of childrens' bodies. A Lund and Browder chart that has precalculated percentages for each body part for different age groups can also be used (Fig. 5.4). For smaller burns, the patient's own hand can be used. The palmer surface has been estimated to be about 1% of the patient's body surface area, but this approach may overestimate burn size.

Assessment of airway involvement includes checking for singed nasal and facial hairs, dysphonia, and stridor, particularly if the burn took place in an enclosed space or if there are head and neck burns. Carbonaceous material may be present in the mouth and upper airway. Direct laryngoscopy and bronchoscopy may be indicated to supplement the diagnosis not only by allowing direct visualization of the upper airway and the tracheobronchial tree, but also by helping to assess edema and need for intubation. The chest radiograph will usually be remarkably normal. Carbon monoxide levels can be measured to assess for poisoning; however, time from exposure and use of supplemental oxygen will affect the interpretation of the value obtained.

Other important issues in the initial evaluation include assessment of the circulation and compartments of circumferentially

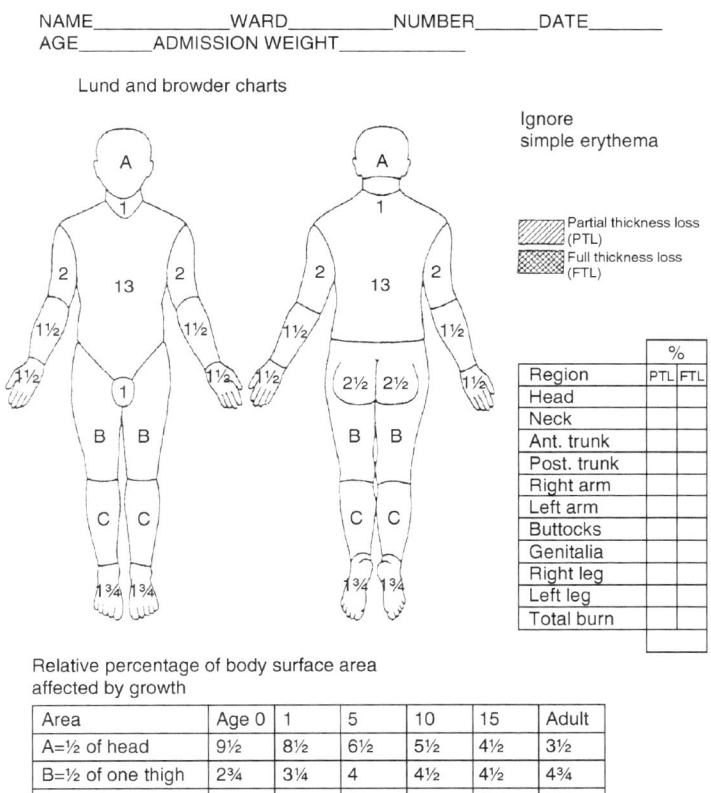

NAME_____WARD_____NUMBER_____DATE_____
AGE_____ADMISSION WEIGHT_____

Lund and browder charts

Ignore
simple erythema

Partial thickness loss
(PTL)
Full thickness loss
(FTL)

	%	
Region	PTL	FTL
Head		
Neck		
Ant. trunk		
Post. trunk		
Right arm		
Left arm		
Buttocks		
Genitalia		
Right leg		
Left leg		
Total burn		

Relative percentage of body surface area
affected by growth

Area	Age 0	1	5	10	15	Adult
A=½ of head	9½	8½	6½	5½	4½	3½
B=½ of one thigh	2¾	3¼	4	4½	4½	4¾
C=½ of one leg	2½	2½	2¾	3	3¼	3½

FIGURE 5.4. An example of a Lund and Browder chart used for assessment of % TBSA burn.

burned limbs and limbs involved in the pathway of electrical injury. Pulses, capillary refill, temperature, swelling, movement, and sensation should be documented. A full neurologic exam should be undertaken. In electrical injuries, an electrocardiogram is imperative, the patient should be monitored for 24 h, and urine checked for myoglobin. Baseline blood gas, electrolyte, and hematologic values are obtained.

The possibility of non-accidental injury in pediatric thermal injuries must remain in the healthcare workers mind. Suspicious findings in the history include an evasive or changing story, a delay in seeking medical help, a story that does not fit with the age of the child or the pattern of injury, or lack of adequate supervision at the time of injury. There may be evidence of a "tide-line" and sparing of the flexion creases in an immersion type injury where the burn lines up when the child goes into the fetal position. Also, glove and stocking type injuries to hands and feet, deep contact burns, e.g. with an iron pattern, and no splash marks in a scald injury should arouse suspicion. Other injuries or evidence of past injuries and signs of neglect should be sought, and careful photography and documentation of the case undertaken. The child should be admitted to the hospital until the case can be assessed by the relevant authorities.

Treatment

First aid for a thermal injury consists of removing the victim from the source of injury in a manner that does not cause harm to the rescuer. Ignited clothing should be extinguished by getting the victim to drop to the ground and roll. Wet blankets can also be used. The clothing should then be removed. Electrical power sources should be sought and turned off before attempting to help the victim. Cooling measures should then be applied, such as running cool or lukewarm water. Very cold water or ice should be avoided because the blood flow to the burned area may be decreased, and the victim may become hypothermic.

The initial management of a major burn then follows that of a trauma patient with assessment of the ABCs, i.e., airway, breathing, circulation, as well as the cervical spine. Supplemental oxygen should be provided. If signs of inhalation injury are present or facial or neck burns are present, airway patency should be assessed. Stridor or other signs of acute respiratory distress indicate need for intubation. If a bronchoscopy is being done to evaluate the airway, an endotracheal tube can be passed over the scope and the patient intubated if necessary. Patients at risk for progressive edema, but without significant swelling, can be observed for 24–36 h; however, in established edema, intubation can be very difficult. Once a secure airway has been established, breathing needs to be re-assessed. In circumferential, full-thickness chest burns, ventilation may be impaired due to the reduced chest wall compliance. Chest wall escharotomies can improve ventilation substantially in these patients.

Circulation then needs to be assessed. Vital signs and urine output are monitored and intravenous access obtained. The depth and % TBSA burn should be calculated and the need for intravenous resuscitation assessed. In general, burns over 15% TBSA require intravenous fluid resuscitation (Hettiaratchy and Dziewulski, 2004). Several formulae have been used to try and establish the correct amount and type of resuscitative fluid. One of the most commonly used calculations is the Parkland formula which uses lactated Ringers solution at a rate of 3–4 ml/kg body weight/% TBSA burn, which gives the 24 h fluid requirement from the time of burn; half is to be given in the first 8 h post burn, and the remaining half given over the next 16 h. Children require dextrose-containing maintenance fluids in addition when using this formula. The use of colloid versus crystalloid in acute burn resuscitation has been long debated. Proponents of colloid argue that the reduced volumes required minimize the cardiac and electrolyte complications of infusion of large volumes of fluid; however, the benefit of colloid has not been proven in the first 24 h post burn. Regardless of the formula used, the calculation should serve as a general guideline to the amount of fluid needed, and end-points of resuscitation need to be monitored. Some patients may need more fluid and some may need less. Pulse, blood pressure, and urine output are the traditional values monitored (Sheridan, 2000). In children, urine outputs of 1–2 ml/kg/h are desired, while in adults 0.5–1 ml/kg/h is sufficient. Early resuscitation appears to improve outcome.

In full-thickness circumferential burns to the limbs, if there is any impairment to circulation, escharotomies are needed. The incisions should stretch the full range of the burn wound to the edge of normal skin. Generally incisions down each side of the limb are necessary and can usually be performed at the bedside. The fascial compartments should be assessed and, if necessary, also released. In electrical injuries or victims with additional trauma, there should be a lower threshold for fasciotomies. The limbs should be elevated to help reduce further swelling from the resultant edema formation. A secondary survey should be done to assess for any additional injuries, and these treated. Tetanus prophylaxis should be administered if indicated. Early resuscitation and enteral feeding is safe, effective, and important in providing nutrition (Barrow, 2000). Meticulous pulmonary hygiene should be maintained.

For chemical injuries, contaminated clothing should be removed and the area copiously and repeatedly irrigated. Litmus paper may be used to test the pH of the skin to confirm removal of the substance. It is important to know the agent involved, because some chemicals have more specific therapies; for instance, hydrofluoric acid sequesters calcium and calcium gluconate should be applied topically or injected locally. Systemic administration may also be necessary. Eye injuries should also be irrigated copiously and a fluorescein stain done to check for corneal abrasions. If any injury is suspected, the patient should be referred to an ophthalmologist.

Superficial partial-thickness wounds generally do not require operation and are treated topically. A wide variety of dressings are available and suitable for use. The wounds need to be cleaned first and then the dressing applied. Paraffin gauze or hydrocolloid dressings are suitable for clean, superficial wounds. Traditionally, silver-containing ointments and soaks, such as silver sulfadiazine and silver nitrate have also been used. The silver imparts bactericidal properties to the ointments. Biobrane, a bilaminar silicone membrane bonded to a collagen layer, can be applied to these types of wounds because it adheres to the wound, reduces pain and the need for dressing changes, and has good quality healing results. This agent needs to be monitored initially for adherence and infection, and should be removed if not sticking or infected.

Human amnion membrane has also been used successfully in treatment of partial-thickness burns, although it carries a potential risk of transmission of infectious diseases (Sheridan, 2000). Numerous other topical dressings and ointments are also available.

Deeper burn wounds require operative treatment. Deep dermal injuries may be treated by debriding the wound tangentially to healthy bleeding tissue. If a significant portion of the dermis is still intact, the wound may be covered temporarily with porcine xenograft or human allograft. If the dermis re-epithelializes, the xeno- or allograft will gradually lift off. If not, it will have to be removed at a later procedure and the area autografted with split-thickness skin grafts taken from the patient's available unburned skin. Full-thickness wounds require complete excision of the dermis. If the subcutaneous tissue underneath is also burned or infected, it may be necessary to excise the wound to the level of fascia. Again, split-thickness autograft is the coverage of choice for these patients. The graft is usually harvested at a depth of 8–12/1000 in. and is not usually meshed for facial burns and, if possible, for hand burns. Otherwise, the graft is usually meshed to allow for greater coverage and drainage of fluid. In large burns, often there is insufficient donor sites to achieve full coverage with autograft in one operation, and multiple debridement and grafting procedures are necessary. The excised wound may be covered temporarily with skin substitutes such as porcine xenograft, human allograft, or synthetic dermal substitutes such as Integra. As the donor sites heal, the burn wounds are autografted serially. Thorough wound care is necessary to reduce the incidence of wound sepsis. Antibiotic therapy should be tailored according to evidence of infection and wound cultures and sensitivities.

It is now possible to use a small sample of unburned skin to culture keratinocytes into epithelial sheets. This approach is most efficacious to cover the patient with very large burns. Problems associated with this approach include fragility of the grafts, delay in obtaining the finished product, and the prohibitive expense for many centers.

Post-operatively, the patient usually requires extensive rehabilitation involving physical therapy to maintain range of motion, the use of splints to prevent joint contractures, and meticulous wound care and scar management. This aspect of therapy is vital and will influence the extent of reconstructive procedures necessary at later stages, such as joint contracture releases. Major burns usually require multiple reconstructive procedures once stable wound coverage has been achieved, including releases of joint contractures and ectropions and reconstruction of destroyed body parts. Moisturization of the healed areas and protection from the sun are also very important.

Outcome

The prognosis for those with thermal injuries has improved over the last 2 decades. Due to advances in techniques of resuscitation, infection control, critical care, and more aggressive surgical management, the mortality for severe burns has decreased markedly. Early fluid resuscitation (commencing within two hours of injury) may have important implications in improving survival and in reducing the incidence of multiorgan failure. The advent of skin substitutes and development of cultured keratinocytes has also improved outcome, because these newer biologic dressings allow better opportunities to achieve wound coverage in large burns. Extremes of age and % TBSA involvement remain important predictors of mortality.

Survival is not the only relevant outcome in thermal injury. Functional outcome, quality of life, participation in society and the work force, and psychologic well-being are all important factors to consider when assessing outcome in the thermally injured patient. Many patients have functional disabilities relating to scar contractures or undergo amputations secondary to burn injuries which impact on activities of daily living and participation in work and school. Patients may become depressed as a result of loss of independence, the necessity to alter their lifestyles, and the alteration in their physical appearances. Psychologic counseling and family and community support are important.

Selected Readings

Atiyeh BS, Gunn SW, Hayek SN (2005) State of the art in burn treatment. World J Surg 29:131–148

Barrow RE, Jeschke MG, Herndon DN (2000) Early fluid resuscitation improves outcomes in severely burned children. Resuscitation 45:91–96

Benson A, Dickson WA, Boyce D (2006) ABC of wound healing. Burns. BMJ 332:649–652

Demling RH (2005) The burn edema process: current concepts. J Burn Care Rehabil 26:207–227

Hettiaratchy S, Dziewulski P (2004) ABC of burns. Pathophysiology and types of burns. BMJ 328:1427–1429 Sheridan RL (2000) Airway management and respiratory care of the burn patient. Int Anesthesiol Clin 38:129–145

Sheridan RL, Tompkins RG (2004) What's new in burns and metabolism. J Am Coll Surg 198:243–263 van Baar M, Essink-Bot ML, Oen IMMH, et al. (2006) Functional outcome after burns: a review. Burns 32:1–9

6
Closed Head Injury

Philip F. Stahel and Wade R. Smith

Pearls and Pitfalls

- Closed head injury represents the leading cause of death in young patients in industrialized countries.
- Patients surviving the initial injury are susceptible to sustaining secondary cerebral insults initiated by the release of endogenous neurotoxic inflammatory mediators.
- Hypoxia and hypotension in the early resuscitative period represents the "key" parameter for induction of secondary brain injury and adverse outcomes.
- The neuroinflammatory response in the injured brain contributes to cerebral edema, increased intracranial pressure (ICP), and decreased cerebral perfusion pressure (CPP).
- ICP monitoring and CPP therapy are recommended as a standard for patients with severe closed head injury. The ICP should be kept below 15 mmHg and the CPP above 70 mmHg in order to avoid secondary insults due to cerebral hypoperfusion.
- If a CPP ≥ 70 mmHg cannot be achieved by lowering the ICP, the mean arterial pressure (MAP) should be artificially raised by the use of catecholamines (CPP = MAP – ICP).
- Arterial "demand" hypertension in head-injured patients should not be lowered therapeutically since this physiological response is aimed at maintaining an adequate CPP once the cerebrovascular autoregulation has failed.

K.I. Bland et al. (eds.), *Trauma Surgery*,
DOI 10.1007/978-1-84996-375-6_6,
© Springer-Verlag London Limited 2011

Common Errors of Practice

- Delayed resuscitation from hypotension and hypoxemia.
- Delayed endotracheal intubation in patients with a Glasgow Coma Scale (GCS) score ≤ 8.
- Lack of attention to associated injuries (thoracic, abdominal, orthopedic).
- Underestimating magnitude of mild or moderate head injury, assuming absence of intracranial pathology (patients who "talk and die").
- Underestimating comatose patients with normal computed tomography (CT) scan (diffuse axonal injury).
- Failures in awake patients: (1) Inadequate frequency of neurological examinations; (2) delay in obtaining a CT scan upon neurological deterioration or change in pupil size/reactivity.
- Pharmacological attenuation of increased systemic blood pressure in head-injured patients ("demand hypertension").
- "Blind" therapeutic hyperventilation without keeping the pCO_2 in constant range (3.3–4.7 kPa) and without bedside jugular bulb oxymetry and sequential measurement of the arterio-jugular differences in lactate concentrations.
- Delay in transfer of severely head-injured patients to a facility with neurosurgical capabilities.

Introduction

In industrialized nations, closed head injury represents the leading cause of death and disability in young people. In the USA alone, about 1.5–1.8 million people sustain a traumatic brain injury each year, of which approximately 500,000 require hospital admission. The annual economic burden of direct and indirect costs for traumatic brain injury in the USA is estimated around US\$50 billion annually. Despite advances in research and improved neurointensive care in the last decade, the clinical outcome of severely head-injured patients is still poor and the mortality rate remains as high as 35–40%. Research efforts in the past years have highlighted that the intracerebral inflammatory response in the injured brain contributes to the neuropathological sequelae which are, in large part, responsible for the adverse outcome after closed head injury. The extent of residual brain damage is determined by primary and secondary insults. The primary damage results from mechanical forces applied to skull and brain at the time of impact, leading to either focal or diffuse brain injury patterns. Focal brain injury is due to direct concussion/compression forces, while diffuse axonal shearing injuries are usually caused by indirect trauma mechanisms, such as sudden deceleration or rotational acceleration. Secondary brain injury occurs after the initial trauma and is a consequence of complicating processes such as ischemia/reperfusion injuries, cerebral edema, intracranial hemorrhage, and intracranial hypertension. The main risk factors for developing secondary brain injury are hypoxemia and systemic hypotension which occur frequently in the polytraumatized patient. The general surgeon who sees brain-injured patients first, must be skilled in their initial assessment and resuscitation, as a neurosurgeon may not be immediately available. The maintenance of adequate systemic blood pressure and oxygenation is of paramount importance. This chapter provides a concise protocol for the initial assessment and management of patients with closed head injuries.

Clinical Presentation

The diagnosis of closed head injury is established by the history of trauma, by the clinical status, and by CT Scan. Efforts should be made to learn the details of the accident, including the mechanism of trauma. This includes blunt vs. penetrating injury, force of the traumatic impact, condition of the vehicle, and presence of other injured/dead occupants. The condition of the vehicle's interior may reveal potential associated injury patterns, such as a "bull's eye"-break on the windscreen, suggesting direct skull impact with associated shear forces to brain tissue and possibility of associated cervical spine injury, or a bent steering wheel may indicate severe chest trauma leading to hypoxia. The likelihood of serious injuries is significantly increased in patients that have been ejected from the vehicle or in the case of death by another occupant in the same vehicle compartment. It is furthermore important to obtain information about the level of consciousness at the accident scene, the presence of impaired neurologic function, and changes in the level of consciousness until admission to the hospital. Of particular importance is the knowledge of the postresuscitation GCS score, since this parameter represents an important predictor of outcome (Table 6.1). Other crucial information includes the presence of anoxia/hypoxia (compromised airways, chest trauma, delayed endotracheal intubation) and the approximate blood loss at the accident scene (massive external bleeding, hemorrhagic shock), as well as the therapy instituted before admission (airway patency, endotracheal intubation, adequate fluid resuscitation).

On the accident scene and on hospital admission, all head-injured patients must be systemically assessed and resuscitated according to the American College of Surgeons' "Advanced Trauma Life Support" (ATLS) protocol. The recommendations for the initial management of patients with closed head injury are presented in > Table 6.2. After securing the airway and assuring adequate oxygenation and fluid replacement, concomitant intra-abdominal injuries leading to exsanguinating hemorrhage must be excluded in all head-injured patients with an altered level of consciousness by ultrasonography and/or CT scan. Furthermore, an associated cervical spine injury must be assumed in all head-injured patients until proven otherwise, since 5–10% of head-injured patients have concomitant injuries of the cervical spine. The neurologic evaluation is initiated only after vital functions have been stabilized. The level of consciousness is rapidly assessed by the GCS score (Table 6.1). When assessing the GCS, the best response post resuscitation is used to calculate the score. In addition to the level of consciousness, the neurologic exam must include the assessment of pupillary

TABLE 6.1. Glasgow Outcome Scale (GOS) (Jennett and Bond, 1975).

Clinical parameter	Points
Eye opening (E)	
Spontaneous	4
To speech	3
To pain	2
None	1
BEST motor response (M)	
Obeys commands	6
Localizes pain	5
Normal flexion (withdrawal)	4
Abnormal flexion (decorticate)	3
Extension (decerebrate)	2
None (flaccid)	1
Verbal response (V)	
Fully oriented	5
Disoriented/confused conversation	4
Inappropriate words	3
Incomprehensible words	2
None	1
GCS score: Σ (E + M + V)	Severity of head injury
14/15 points	Mild
9–13 points	Moderate
3–8 points	Severe

size and reactivity, and a brief focused evaluation of peripheral motor function. The clinical exam furthermore includes the inspection of the scalp for lacerations, palpation of the skull for impression fractures, and the search for indirect signs of basilar skull fractures, including periorbital ecchymosis

TABLE 6.2. Initial management of head-injured patients (*see text for details and abbreviations*) (Stahel et al., 2005; The Brain Trauma Foundation, 2006).

- Initial assessment and resuscitation according to the ATLS protocol. Secure airways and assure adequate oxygenation and fluid replacement. Avoid hypoxemia and hypotension!

- Exclude exsanguinating intra-abdominal injury (focused ultrasonography/"FAST," CT) and other associated systemic injuries.

- Blood alcohol level and urine toxic screening in all head-injured patients.

- *History*:

  – Mechanism and time of injury

  – Loss of consciousness

  – Amnesia (retro-/anterograde)

  – Postresuscitation level of consciousness (GCS)

  – Seizures

  – Presence of headache (mild/moderate/severe)

- *Brief neurologic examination*:

  – Level of consciousness (GCS)

  – Pupillary size and reaction

  – Focal motor deficits

- Indications for CT scan:

  – All patients with moderate to severe head injury (GCS < 14).

  – Mild head injury (GCS 14 and 15) in conjunction with one of the following criteria:

    – Presence of skull fracture (clinically or xray)

    – CSF leak (rhinorrhea, otorrhea)

    – Alcohol/drug intoxication

    – Moderate to severe headache

    – Focal neurologic deficits, abnormal pupil size or reactivity

    – Deteriorating level of consciousness (GCS < 14) in the later course

(continued)

TABLE 6.2   (continued)

> – Perform a control CT scan before discharge in all patients with moderate to severe head injury (GCS < 14) and in cases of mild head injury (GCS 14 and 15) with pathological initial CT scan.

- *Indications for hospital admission*:

  - All patients with GCS < 15 (observe for at least 24 h, with frequent neurologic examinations)

  - All patients with open head injuries, CSF leak, skull fractures

  - Patients with GCS 15 and one of the following: (1) moderate to severe headache; (2) history of loss of consciousness; (3) amnesia; (4) significant alcohol/drug intoxication; (5) no reliable companion at home for observation; (6) unable to return promptly in case of deterioration.

("raccoon eyes"), retroauricular ecchymosis ("Battle's sign"), rhinorrhea/otorrhea due to cerebrospinal fluid (CSF) leakage, and VIIth nerve palsy. The necessity for obtaining a CT scan (Table 6.2) is given under the following circumstances: (1) altered level of consciousness; (2) abnormal neurologic examination; (3) differences in pupil size or reactivity; (4) suspected skull fracture. Furthermore, the CT scan should be repeated whenever there is deterioration in the patient's neurologic status.

Classification

Closed head injury may be classified either by morphology, severity, or mechanism of injury. The morphological classification is based on findings in the CT scan according to the guidelines established by Marshall and colleagues (Fig. 6.1). Intracranial CT lesions can be either of focal nature ("evacuated" vs. "non-evacuated" subdural, epidural, or intracerebral hematomas) or diffuse (grade I–IV). The classification by severity according to the GCS score (Table 6.1) is clinically relevant, since the postresuscitation score has been shown to significantly correlate with patient outcome. Patients with mild

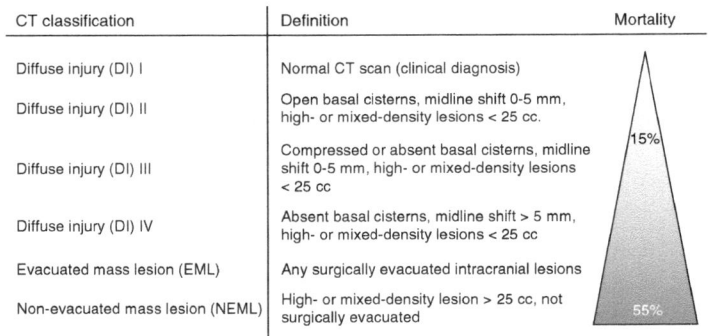

CT classification	Definition	Mortality
Diffuse injury (DI) I	Normal CT scan (clinical diagnosis)	
Diffuse injury (DI) II	Open basal cisterns, midline shift 0-5 mm, high- or mixed-density lesions < 25 cc.	
Diffuse injury (DI) III	Compressed or absent basal cisterns, midline shift 0-5 mm, high- or mixed-density lesions < 25 cc	15%
Diffuse injury (DI) IV	Absent basal cisterns, midline shift > 5 mm, high- or mixed-density lesions < 25 cc	
Evacuated mass lesion (EML)	Any surgically evacuated intracranial lesions	
Non-evacuated mass lesion (NEML)	High- or mixed-density lesion > 25 cc, not surgically evacuated	55%

FIGURE 6.1. Morphological classification by CT scan. The classification of intracranial pathology by CT scan according to Marshall et al. correlates significantly with the outcome after closed head injury (Marshall et al., 1992).

head injury (GCS 14 or 15) represent about 80% of all head-trauma patients admitted to the emergency department. These patients usually suffer from a mild cerebral concussion which corresponds to diffuse brain injury with preserved consciousness but a certain degree of temporary neurologic dysfunction. In contrast, a "classic" cerebral concussion results in a reversible loss of consciousness, which is always accompanied by posttraumatic amnesia. It is important to keep in mind that approximately 3% of patients with *mild* head injury will have a potentially fatal intracranial hemorrhage. Thus, all patients with closed head injury should be admitted to the hospital according to the recommendations outlined in Table 6.2. Pitfall: Patients who "talk and die" comprise those who have a GCS > 8 on admission and suddenly deteriorate due to an intracranial mass lesion, typically an acute epidural hematoma (EDH).

Moderate head injury corresponds to a GCS score between 9 and 13 and is associated with an increased risk for intracranial pathology compared to patients with *mild* head injury. As outlined in Table 6.2, a CT scan must be performed in all patients with *moderate* head injury, and all of these patients should be admitted to the hospital for observation. A GCS score ≤ 8 corresponds to a comatose patient, as defined by the inability to open the eyes, to obey commands, and to respond verbally. Thus, *severe* head injury is defined as a GCS score of 3–8. The initial assessment and management of these severely injured patients is described in the following section.

Emergency Room Management

The immediate goal in the management of head-injured patients is the prevention of secondary brain damage by rapid correction of hypoxemia, hypotension, hypercarbia, and hypoglycemia. For airway protection, an oropharyngeal or nasopharyngeal airway may be adequate in drowsy patients with sufficient breathing, while endotracheal intubation by "rapid sequence induction" is indicated in comatose patients (GCS ≤ 8) or in cases of apnea, hypoventilation, risk of upper airway obstruction (maxillofacial fractures, laryngeal injury), and aspiration (vomiting, bleeding). Adequate volume resuscitation is crucial, including the control of external and internal hemorrhages. According to the ATLS guidelines, the initial fluid therapy should be an isotonic electrolyte solution, such as Ringer's lactate, with an initial bolus dose of 1,000–2,000 ml in adults and 20 ml/kg in children. Measurement of the urinary output represents a "prime monitor" for the patients' response to resuscitation, and should be about 0.5 ml/kg/h in adults and 1–2 ml/kg/h in pediatric patients. Pitfall: Increased urinary output in head-injured patients due to syndrome of inappropriate ADH secretion (SIADH). A detailed neurologic evaluation should only be initiated after the vital systems have been stabilized. Furthermore, associated injuries, such as a cervical spine injury, blunt chest trauma, intra-abdominal injuries, pelvic ring disruptions, and open fractures must receive adequate attention, as all of these injuries can potentiate the extent of secondary brain damage. According to the ATLS algorithm for early care of severely injured patients, the "A-B-C-D-E" priorities mandate

Box 6.1 Relationship between CPP, ICP and MAP[a]

CPP = MAP – ICP

[a]CPP, cerebral perfusion pressure; ICP, intracranial pressure; MAP, mean arterial pressure.

that only hemodynamically stable patients should undergo further diagnostics, such as a craniocerebral CT scan. All head-injured patients with presence of hypoxia and/or hypotension must be fully resuscitated, if required by surgical measures, before CT diagnostics are performed.

The main priority in the early management of head-trauma patients is the maintenance of an adequate CPP above 70–80 mmHg. According to the "Monro-Kellie doctrine," the total intracranial volume remains constant, implying that expanding mass lesions will result in a reduced CPP, thus contributing to secondary brain injury. Due to the interrelation between CPP and MAP (Box 6.1), an increased systemic blood pressure must never be therapeutically lowered in head-injured patients unless continuous ICP-monitoring is available ("demand" hypertension!). Standardized therapeutic approaches are aimed at lowering the ICP in order to keep the CPP at a sufficient level. Among the therapeutic modalities are the reduction of mass lesions by surgical evacuation of intracranial hematomas (ICHs), the reduction of brain swelling with osmotic drugs, e.g., mannitol, and therapeutic CSF drainage through intraventricular catheters.

Osmotic Therapy (Mannitol)

When given as a bolus, mannitol augments the intravascular volume, resulting in a transient increase in MAP and CPP. Mannitol also causes an increase in cerebral blood flow (CBF) in cases of impaired cerebrovascular autoregulation, where CBF is directly dependent on systemic arterial pressure.

Furthermore, mannitol can induce a cerebral vasoconstriction, resulting in a diminished intracranial volume.

Indications:

- Clinical signs of transtentorial herniation (i.e., loss of consciousness, decerebrate rigidity, ipsilateral pupil dilatation, contralateral hemiparesis), or progressive neurological deterioration, not attributable to systemic pathology.
- Bilaterally dilated and nonreactive pupils.
- Regimen: mannitol (20%), 0.25–1 g/kg IV in 5 min.

Pitfalls:

- Hypovolemia must be avoided by adequate fluid replacement.
- Serum osmolarity must be kept <315 mOsm/l, since hyperosmolarity may induce acute renal failure.

The use of *glucocorticoids* is not recommended for attenuating the neuroinflammatory response in severely head-injured patients. In contrast, based on the devastating results from the prospective multicenter "CRASH" trial on 10,008 head-injured patients randomized for high-dose methylprednisolone vs. placebo, steroids are now considered harmful for patients with closed head injury as they are associated with a significant increase in posttraumatic mortality. *Barbiturates* are effective in reducing ICP; however, their use is restricted for intensive care therapy with continuous EEG monitoring.

Indications for evacuation of intracranial hematomas:

- Generally, an ICH causing neurological deterioration or >5 mm midline shift in CT scan should be evacuated as soon as possible
- Evacuation of acute subdural hematomas (aSDH) of >3 mm thickness
- Evacuation of aSDH <3 mm in comatose patients with severe parenchymal injuries and mass effect
- For EDH, surgical evacuation is generally indicated, except in clinically stable patients with a small EDH and minimal pathological findings (GCS 14 or 15)

- Evacuation of large ICH in patients with focal neurological deficits and/or a midline shift in CT scan
- Depressed skull fractures: Indication for operative elevation if the extent of depression is thicker than the adjacent skull in CT scan
- Apart from the evacuation of ICHs, all open head injuries represent an indication for neurosurgical intervention

Indications for continuous ICP-monitoring:

- Patients with severe head injury (postresuscitation GCS ≤8) and abnormal admission CT scan
- Patients with severe head injury (GCS ≤8) and normal initial CT scan, but with a prolonged coma >6h
- Patients requiring evacuation of ICHs
- Neurological deterioration (GCS ≤8) in patients with initially mild or moderate head injury
- Head-injured patients requiring prolonged mechanical ventilation, e.g., due to operations for extracranial injuries, unless the initial CT scan is normal

Intraoperative Management

Craniotomy

One third of patients with severe closed head injury need immediate craniotomy for evacuation of mass lesions, most commonly for aSDH. There is a clear benefit to early evacuation of significant intracranial mass lesions. In patients with clinically *mild* or *moderate* brain injury, craniotomy is performed for depressed skull fractures or for "stable" hematomas on a less urgent basis. The timing of surgery depends on the clinical condition of the patient, in particular on the neurologic exam and CT findings. A comatose patient with a significant intracerebral hematoma causing hemispheric shifting should be taken immediately to surgery. Three types of ICH are encountered as surgical removable mass lesions: (1) aSDH from tearing of a bridging vein from the cortex to the venous sinuses or a cortical artery; (2) EDH from laceration of the middle meningeal artery or from the edges of a skull fracture; and (3) ICH from bleeding within the brain parenchyma. A standard craniotomy is performed with the patient supine and the head turned to the appropriate side and fixed in a Mayfield clamp. The incision is started just anterior to the ear and extended superiorly, 2 cm lateral and parallel to the midline, in the shape of a large question mark. A burr hole is made above the ear, which marks the bottom part of the temporal fossa, to allow immediate evacuation in case of EDH, or evacuation of SDH following incision of the dura. Additional burr holes have to be placed approximately 1.5 cm off the midline to avoid injury to major venous structures, such as the sinus sagittalis. Depending on the type of hematoma, a sufficiently large bone flap is performed for adequate exposure. An EDH is removed after elevation of the bone flap and the lacerated vessel has to be identified and cauterized. SDHs and ICHs can be approached after opening of the dura, which has to be lifted off the underlying cortex carefully. The hematoma is then gently evacuated by suction, irrigation, or other mechanical means. The origin of the hematoma must be identified and cauterized. If necessary, parts of contused brain can be debrided. Complete hemostasis must be achieved prior to closure of the dura. If this is not possible, a tamponade may be performed by the use of topical hemostatic agents (e.g., FloSeal) or by autologous muscle interponates. A Valsalva maneuver may be helpful for verification of secure hemostasis. The dura must be sealed tightly, which can be achieved by the use of an artificial dura patch. Dural tack-up sutures are placed around the periphery of the bony exposure and in the center of the flap. Epidural drains are put in place, after which the bone flap is refixed. In cases of expected postoperative brain swelling, it is advisable to postpone the implantation of the bone flap to a later time-point. Under these circumstances, the resected skull can be stored safely at −80C or else implanted subcutaneously into the abdominal wall of the patient. Finally, the temporal fascia, galea, and skin are closed.

Note: Small lesions in the temporal or in the posterior fossa may cause compression to the brainstem and/or obstruction of the CSF flow, therefore early surgical intervention is warranted.

For removal of hematomas in the posterior fossa the patient is operated in a prone position.

Emergency Burr Holes

In areas where neuroradiologic imaging (CT scan)or neurosurgical intervention are not readily available, general surgeons should be knowledgeable about the option of placing cranial burr holes for evacuation of ICHs. *Indication*: Rapidly deteriorating neurologic status, not responsive to osmotic therapy (mannitol); e.g., patients with suspected EDH whose level of consciousness or focal neurologic deficit is acutely worsening. The patient is positioned as described above for a craniotomy. A burr hole is placed on the side of the pupillary dilatation or contralateral to the side of the motor deficit. An incision anterior to the ear is taken down to the os zygomaticum, which marks the bottom of the temporal fossa. The hole may be enlarged for evacuation of an EDH or an SDH, the latter after incision of the dura. If necessary, a complete craniotomy can be performed as an enlargement of this approach.

Pitfalls:

- The majority of comatose patients do not have an ICH which needs to be evacuated
- burr hole may miss the hematoma or drain it insufficiently
- burr hole may itself induce intracranial bleeding
- Placing a burr hole may consume as much time as transferring the patient to a center with neurosurgical capabilities

Management in the ICU

Postoperatively, patients are transferred to intensive care unit (ICU) and treated according to standardized protocols. The goals of ICU therapy are:

- Achievement and maintenance of adequate gas exchange and circulatory stability by means of endotracheal intubation, mechanical ventilation, adequate volume resuscitation, and administration of vasoactive drugs, if required, as well as prevention of hypoxemia and hypercarbia. The goal is to keep PaO2 > 13 kPa and PaCO2 between 3.3 and 4.5 kPa. No "blind" prophylactic hyperventilation, due to the risk of inducing focal ischemic insults. Aggressive circulatory stabilization: MAP > 80 mmHg, normovolemia, hematocrit ≥ 30%.

Note: No antihypertensive therapy up to MAP of 130 mmHg ("demand" hypertension!).

- Repeated, scheduled CT scans for detection of delayed secondary intracranial pathology which may have to be surgically evacuated.
- Profound but easily reversible sedation and analgesia to avoid stress and pain, which may result in increases of ICP and the cerebral metabolic rate.
- Achievement and maintenance of optimal CPP (>70 mmHg) and cerebral oxygen balance, allowing recovery of damaged brain areas and prevention of secondary brain damage. Here, the monitoring tools include (1) frequent blood gas analyses, (2) continuous ICP registration, (3) jugular bulb oximetry, (4) assessment of arterio-jugular difference in lactate concentrations, (5) transcranial Doppler sonography for assessment of CBF/vasospasms, and (6) repeated or continuous EEG registration. Administration of nimodipine in patients with signs of vasospasm detected by Doppler sonography.
- Avoidance of hyperthermia (< 38°C).
- Prevention of hyperglycemia and hyponatremia.
- No routinely performed head elevation (attenuation of CPP!).
- Prevention of stress ulcers and maintenance of gut mucosal integrity by early administration of enteral nutrition.
- Prophylaxis for complicating factors, e.g., pneumonia or meningitis; repeated bacteriological sampling (including CSF through ventricular catheters) and anti-infectious treatment, if necessary.

Therapy in the event of elevated ICP (>15 mmHg, >5 min), after exclusion of surgically removable intracranial mass lesions (step-by-step regimen):

1. Deepening of sedation, analgesia, muscle relaxation.

    - CSF drainage through ventricular catheters, where applicable
    - Moderate hyperventilation, as long as: (a) jugular bulb oxygenation > 60%, (b) arterio-jugular difference in lactate < 0.2 mmol/l, (c) an ICP-lowering effect can be achieved by hyperventilation

2. Osmotherapy: mannitol (20%) bolus IV in steps of 25 – 50 – 100 ml, as long as serum osmolarity < 315 mOsm/l.

3. Moderate hypothermia (± 34°C).

4. Barbiturate coma (thiopental IV) under continuous EEG registration. Goal: Burst suppression pattern of 6 bursts/min and a burst suppression relationship of 1:1.

Complications

General complications of severe head injury:

- Cerebral edema may lead to supratentorial swelling and herniation of the brain through the dural hiatuses and the foramen magnum.
- *Ischemic brain injury*, following brain herniation or focal cerebral vasospasms.
- *Posttraumatic immunosuppression*, leading to increased susceptibility to pulmonary infections, sepsis, and multi-organ failure.
- *Neurogenic pulmonary edema*. Definition: Pulmonary edema after head injury in the absence of cardial or pulmonary disorders or hypervolemia. Pitfall: Fluid overload in brain-injured patients.
- *Syndrome of inappropriate ADH secretion* (SIADH), characterized by hyponatremia, hyposmolarity, and urinary sodium > 25 mEq/l. After hemodynamic stabilization, these patients should be treated by restriction of fluid intake to about 800–1,000 ml/day, using isotonic intravenous fluids (e.g., Ringer's lactate).

- *Disseminated intravascular coagulation* (DIC). The damaged brain tissue represents a powerful activator of the coagulation cascade and may cause a severe consumptive coagulopathy.
- *Gastrointestinal bleeding*. Ulcers of the esophagus, stomach, and duodenum are frequent in comatose head-trauma patients. Prophylaxis: Early enteral nutrition, antacids, and proton pump inhibitors.
- *Heterotopic ossification*. Definition: Late complication of brain injury with unclear etiology, characterized by bone formation in tissues that do not normally ossify. The incidence has been reported in 10–86% of patients with severe head-trauma or spinal cord injury, and represents a major source of morbidity and persisting disability in the course of rehabilitation.

Postoperative complications:

- Incomplete evacuation of intracranial mass lesions
- Reoccurrence of intracranial bleeding
- Surgical infections, e.g., meningitis, meningoencephalitis, brain abscess

Complications of ICU therapy:

- *Cerebral vasospasm* after therapeutic hyperventilation. Prophylaxis: Keeping pCO_2 in constant range (3.3–4.5 kPa) and monitoring of arterio-jugular lactate concentrations, jugular bulb oxymetry, and frequent transcranial Doppler sonography.
- *Complications of Barbiturate coma*: Cardiovascular depression, hepatotoxicity, immunosuppression, and increased incidence of pulmonary infections.

Outcome

The GCS, although originally not intended as a prognostic index, is a strong indicator of outcome after closed head injury. Prospective data from the Traumatic Coma Data Bank (TCDB) in the 1980s revealed that patients with severe head injury (GCS score ≤ 8) had an overall mortality rate of 36% at 6 months post injury. Among these, an initial GCS score of 3 was associated with the highest mortality (76%), compared to patients with a score of 6–8 (18%). Patients with moderate head injury (GCS score 9–13) are at particular risk of intracranial complications, and their overall mortality is about 7%. Interestingly, patients who "talk" at admission (GCS score > 8) and then deteriorate have a significantly higher mortality than patients with an initial score ≤ 8. While mortality represents a parameter of outcome which is easy to define, the residual impairment in terms of neurological, cognitive, or behavioral deficits is more difficult to assess. Numerous tests and scores offer different approaches for determining the posttraumatic neurological and neuropsychological impairment. For example, the Disability Rating Scale (DRS) and the Glasgow Outcome Scale (GOS; > Table 6.4) represent traditional measures of global outcome which provide a basis for comparing the results of treatment in different centers. When analyzed using the GOS, only about 60% of patients with *moderate* head injury have an overall good recovery by 6 months after trauma (GOS score 5), whereas a moderate (GOS score 4) to severe disability (GOS score 3) is described in 26% and 7%, respectively.

TABLE 6.3. Glasgow Outcome Scale (GOS) (Jennett and Bond, 1975).

Outcome (assessed 3 or 6 months after head injury)	Characteristics	Score
Good recovery	Reintegrated	5
Moderate disability	Independent but disabled	4
Severe disability	Conscious but dependent	3
Persistent vegetative state	Wakefulness without awareness	2
Death		1

Analysis of the outcome after *mild* head injury (GCS score 14 or 15) revealed that these patients frequently have post-traumatic neuropsychological sequelae. The likelihood of post-concussional symptoms 1 week after trauma ranged from 80% to 93%, and follow-up studies revealed that up to 60% of patients had residual neurobehavioral deficits after 3 months. However, long-term neurological deficits are rare in patients with *mild* head injury.

Selected Readings

Bayir H, Clark RS, Kochanek PM (2003) Promising strategies to minimize secondary brain injury after head trauma. Crit Care Med 31:S112–S117

Finfer SR, Cohen J (2001) Severe traumatic brain injury. Resuscitation 48:77–90

Gaetz M (2004) The neurophysiology of brain injury. Clin Neurophysiol 115:4–18

Jennett B, Bond M (1975) Assessment of outcome after severe brain damage. Lancet 1 (7905):480–484

Marshall LF, Marshall SB, Klauber MR, et al. (1992) The diagnosis of head injury requires a classification based on computed axial tomography. J Neurotrauma 9 (Suppl. 1): S287–S292

McArthur DL, Chute DJ, Villablanca JP (2004) Moderate and severe traumatic brain injury: epidemiologic, imaging and neuropathologic perspectives. Brain Pathol 14:185–194

Narayan RK, Michel ME, Ansell B, et al. (2002) Clinical trials in head injury. J Neurotrauma 19:503–557

Roberts I, Yates D, Sandercock P, et al. (2004) Effect of intravenous corticosteroids on death within 14 days in 10,008 adults with clinically significant head injury (MRC CRASH trial): randomised placebo-controlled trial. Lancet 364:1321–1328

Schmidt OI, Heyde CE, Ertel W, Stahel PF (2005) Closed head injury: an inflammatory disease? Brain Res Rev 48:388–399

Stahel PF, Heyde CE, Ertel W (2005) Current concepts of polytrauma management. Eur J Trauma 31:200–211

Stover JF, Steiger P, Stocker R (2005) Treating intracranial hypertension in patients with severe traumatic brain injury during neurointensive care: new features of old problems? Eur J Trauma 31:308–330

Teasdale G, Jennett B (1974) Assessment of coma and im-paired consciousness: a practical scale. Lancet 2:81–84

The Brain Trauma Foundation (2006) Guidelines for the management of severe traumatic brain injury, 3rd edn. http://www.braintrauma.org

7
Spinal Trauma

Fritz U. Niethard and Markus Weißkopf

Pearls and Pitfalls

- Principles for the treatment of spinal injuries include reduction of the traumatic spinal dislocation. With reduction, most of the dislocated osteoligamentous tissue is realigned by the ligamentous axis. Additional decompression may thereafter be performed. Finally, the reduced injured tissue is held in place by stabilization.
- The fracture classification for spinal injuries proposed by Magerl et al. is generally accepted for the lower cervical and thoracolumbar spine. This classification is based primarily on both pathologic and morphologic aspects. Three mechanisms of trauma are differentiated: compression, distraction, and rotation.
- Current surgical concepts utilizing state-of-the-art implants enable stability of the injured spine to be regained fully with minor surgical trauma and minimal permanent loss of segmental mobility.
- Overdistraction during reduction maneuvers can lead to additional compromise of neural tissue in cases of spinal cord injury (SCI).
- Fractures of the cervicothoracic junction may be missed in patients in whom appropriate traction is not applied on the shoulder girdle.
- In complete SCI, prognosis for recovery of physiologic motor capabilities remains poor.

K.I. Bland et al. (eds.), *Trauma Surgery*,
DOI 10.1007/978-1-84996-375-6_7,
© Springer-Verlag London Limited 2011

Introduction

The spine must serve various functions. In addition to its static function in maintaining upright posture, the spine facilitates motion of both the head in relation to the chest and the chest in relation to the pelvis. It also serves a protective function for the spinal cord. Injury of the spine will result in the loss of these combined functions. A treatment concept for the restoration of the traumatized spine will thus have to address the **reduction** of dislocated structures, the **decompression** of compromised neural tissue, and the **stabilization** of the affected segments to prevent further injury.

Epidemiology and Socioeconomic Impact

Spinal fractures comprise between 0.5% and 2% of all fractures. L1 and Th12 are the most common site of fractures. The thoracolumbar transition is affected in more than 50% of patients.

In 10–15% of spine injuries, more than one level is affected. Spinal trauma is accompanied in 50–60% of cases by other injuries, and in 25–30% it is combined with polytrauma. In a fall from great height, spinal injuries can be associated with calcaneal and hip fractures. Spinal injuries are often caused by traffic accidents (50%) followed by occupational injuries (20%). The increasing number of high-risk sporting activities (such as hang gliding and parachuting) accounts for 10–15% of spinal injuries. In 6% of cases, spinal trauma is a consequence of attempted suicide. The annual reported incidence rate for spinal cord injury (SCI) varies from 25 to 93 per 1 million in populations in the Western world, which is an increase in recent years. In most cases, SCI is the sequelae of a motor vehicle accident or a fall from great height. In a Dutch study, the direct costs for patients with unstable fractures associated with neurologic deficits were calculated at an average of €31,900. This cost does not include the expenses that arise out of rehabilitation programs, which are exceptionally high in paraplegic patients.

Initial Treatment

The prognosis of spinal injury is affected frequently by the initial management of the area of trauma. Because of the high coincidence with other injuries, spinal trauma must always be taken into consideration on the initial assessment. Contusion, hematoma, skin abrasions, gibbus formation, and irregular alignment of the spinous processes might serve as external indicators for spinal injuries. Both the report of pain and the provocation of pain on percussion or compression of the spine also point to violation of the spine. An initial neurologic examination provides information about the level of injury. During the resuscitation of the patient, continuous traction should be applied to the spine. Multilevel support is provided by forklift handling in order to warrant an en bloc carriage (Fig. 7.1). The victim is transported on a vacuum mattress, and the C-spine is immobilized in a hard cervical collar (stiff neck). Reduction maneuvers should be avoided outside the hospital. In case of suspected SCI, administration of high-dose methylprednisolone should be initiated outside the hospital.

Corticosteroid Therapy

The effect of high-dose administration of corticosteroids on acute spinal injury was investigated in a randomized, multicenter study. Patients treated with corticosteroids had a significantly better recovery in incomplete spinal injury if the medication was administered immediately after the trauma (within the first 8 h). In more recent reports, the positive effect of the corticosteroid therapy was not confirmed in incomplete cervical SCI; however, administering the dosage regimen is generally recommended, which is given in Table 7.1 in incomplete SCI or in any case of neurologic deterioration.

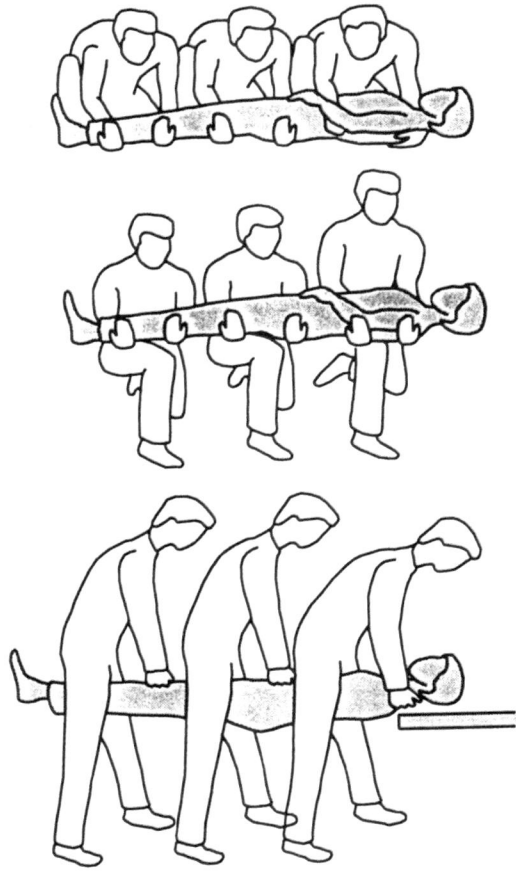

FIGURE 7.1. Initial axis-stable salvage of the trauma victim is performed by an even strain on the various parts of the spine provided by several man support.

TABLE 7.1. Corticosteroid dosage for acute spinal cord injuries.

Dosage	Time interval
30 mg/kg body weight	During 15 min
Pause	For 45 min
5.4 mg/ kg body weight	During 23 h

Diagnostics

During the initial assessment of the patient, it is most important to take a detailed history, because the exact analysis of the mechanism of trauma might be suggestive of associated spinal trauma. On physical examination, the origin of pain origin and external signs of trauma are evaluated in order to localize the injury more precisely. The precise neurologic workup is helpful in determining the exact level of trauma. Early detection of neurologic deficits is of utmost importance, because immediate decompression of the neural structures is the only chance for recovery.

Diagnostic Imaging

Conventional Radiographs

In polytraumatized patients, it is generally recommended to perform x-rays of the C-spine in two planes in addition to anterior–posterior (AP) images of the chest and the pelvis. During the acquisition of the C-spine images, traction is applied to the arms in order to visualize completely the seventh cervical vertebrae. For the assessment of the facet joints, a 15° oblique view, and for the depiction of the neural foramen, a 45° oblique view of the C-spine are performed. The odontoid process can be demonstrated clearly by means of a transorally focused image. The exact course of an odontoid process fracture line can be determined on computed tomography (CT) with films that include sagittal reformations or conventional tomography. Besides traumatization of the bony structures, attention must be directed toward signs of discoligamentous injury, such as:

- Step formation or irregularities in the posterior alignment of the vertebrae
- Altered height of the disk space

- Unequivalent distance of the spinous processes
- Prevertebral shadow formation

Discoligamentous injuries can be displayed more distinctively on functional flexion/extension x-rays. This investigation depends on the patient's compliance and thus may be difficult to carry out in an acutely injured patient with altered mental status. The guided motion is performed by the physician in order to exclude muscle contraction during the maneuver. The standard, conventional radiographic investigation in the region of the thoracic and lumbar spine consists of AP and lateral images. Besides the aspects that refer to the C-spine, the following criteria should be recognized for the thoracic and lumbar spine:

- Angle of the end plates
- Comparison of the anterior and posterior wall height
- Broadening of the vertebrae
- Irregularities or asymmetries of the pedicles
- Misalignment of the vertebrae's axis

Traumatic spondylolysis can be depicted best on oblique views (45°) of the lumbar spine, where the fracture line is visualized in the interarticular portion of the vertebral arch.

Computed Tomography

CT is now part of diagnostic standard in the workup of the spinal trauma patient, particularly those suspected of having spinal injury. CT is of special importance in the assessment of the spinal canal, the stability of the posterior wall, the integrity of the vertebral arch, and the congruence of the facet joints. For a better visualization of rotational spine injuries, the acquired data can be illustrated in 2D and 3D reformations. Currently, it is possible to reduce the data acquisition time with modern scanners to less than 1 min for the whole lumbar spine. Thus, CT is well-suited for the initial acute diagnostic steps.

Magnetic Resonance Imaging

The main advantage of magnetic resonance imaging (MRI) is the optimal illustration of soft tissue structures. Because MRI weighs the water content of different tissues, traumatized tissue will have altered signals because of the edema. In the T2-weighted sequences, edematous tissues appear as an increased signal. Edema, hematomas, and ruptures in the spinal marrow, the intervertebral disk, the longitudinal ligaments, and muscle structures can be demonstrated most sensitively. The T1 sequences illustrate the exact anatomic relationships. For example, the extent of a disk protrusion can be better evaluated using these sequences. Because of the relatively long data acquisition time, this diagnostic media is reserved for the period after vital signs are stabilized.

Biomechanics and Classification of Spinal Injuries

Proper treatment of spinal injuries is initiated based on classification of injury in order to assess the severity of the trauma and thus the resulting instability. Because both rotational and translational motions along the ordinate axis are physiologic, a subtle analysis of the direction of pathologic instability has to be performed. According to biomechanical aspects which are considered in the current classifications, the spine is subdivided into an anterior and a posterior column. The anterior column consists of the vertebral body, the intervertebral disks, and the anterior longitudinal spinal ligament. The posterior column consists of the vertebral arch, the adjacent processes, and all the ligaments including the posterior longitudinal spinal ligament. Compressive load is carried mainly by the anterior column (80%), while the posterior column absorbs 20% of the weight forces. The posterior column has predominately a tension-banding effect, which is maintained by the ligaments and paravertebral muscles. The integrity of the posterior wall of the vertebral bodies has a central importance for the stability of the fracture, because it acts as a fulcrum for the posterior tensile forces. It is of utmost importance to consider these biomechanical relationships in the treatment of spinal injuries, because the decision on whether operative treatment is necessary depends primarily on the stability of the anterior column. In the assessment of the injury direction, the extent and the nature of the instability (i.e., bone and/or soft tissue trauma) has to be defined.

Due to anatomic and functionally different features of the upper and lower C-spine, the classification of the upper C-spine has to be discerned from rest of the spine. There are multiple injury classification schemes published for the upper C-spine addressing the occipito-atlantal and the atlanto-axial joint complex including the concerned vertebrae. Their description would be beyond the scope of this textbook; however, the fracture classification of Anderson and D'Alonso addressing the odontoid process is reported, because this injury is the most common traumatic lesion of the upper spine. Their classification is subdivided into three different types according to the location of the fracture line (Fig. 7.2). Type-II injury is unstable and must be fixed operatively in order to prevent pseudarthrosis, whereas the other fractures can be treated conservatively after closed reduction. In the mid-1990s, a comprehensive fracture classification for the thoracolumbar spine was proposed by Magerl et al. This classification was adopted later for the lower C-spine because of similarities in the functional and biomechanical aspects.

The Magerl classification is based on both pathologic and morphologic criteria with regard to the main mechanism of injury. Spinal trauma is divided into three main groups (A, B, and C) according to their severity. Type-C injury is most unstable. Compression injuries of the vertebral body are classified as Type-A lesions. Type-B injuries are lesions where distraction acts on the anterior and posterior elements of the spine. Spinal trauma where the main force is the axial torque leading to rotational injuries is also rated as a Type-C injury (Fig. 7.3). Further subdivision of these injuries is given in Table 7.2.

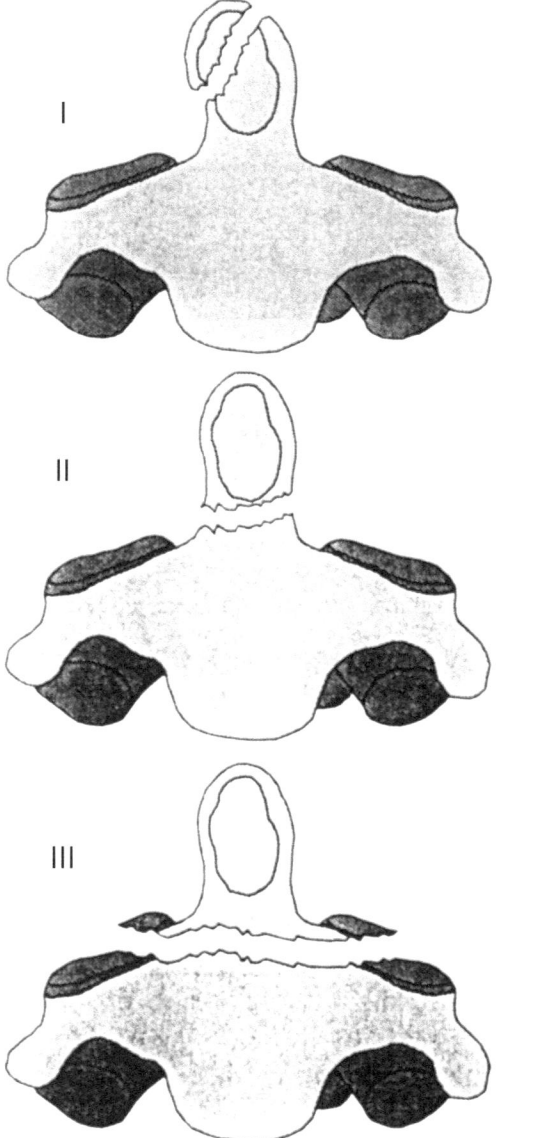

FIGURE 7.2. Odontoid process fracture classification according to Anderson and D'Alonzo.

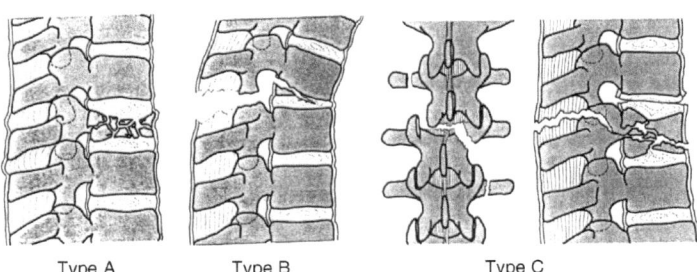

Type A   Type B   Type C

FIGURE 7.3. Various sketches of the Magerl fracture classification for injuries of the thoracolumbar spine.

TABLE 7.2. Classification of spinal injuries after Magerl et al.

Type A: vertebral body compression	Type B: anterior and posterior element injuries with distraction	Type C: anterior and posterior element injuries with rotation
A1: Impaction fracture	B1: Posterior disruption predominantly ligamentous	C1: Type-A injury with rotation
A2: Split fracture	B2: Posterior disruption predominantly osseus	C2: Type-B injury with rotation
A3: Burst fracture	B3: Anterior disruption through the disc	C3: Rotational-shear injuries

Treatment

The general treatment strategy consists of three steps:

- Reduction
- Decompression
- Stabilization

Reduction may be performed as a closed maneuver after the injury is analyzed and classified exactly. According to the instability of the trauma or a possible neurologic deficit, it has to be decided whether a surgical decompression and stabilization is necessary.

Conservative Treatment

Stable injuries of the C-spine generally need no operative intervention. Neck distortions, isolated fracture of the transverse spinous process, or fractures of the apex of the odontoid process (Type I after Anderson and D'Alonso) can be managed as stable injuries and can be treated with a collar. Certain fractures of the base of the odontoid process (Type III after Anderson and D'Alonso) and isolated minor dislocated fractures of the vertebral arch remain stable under tension and compression. In contrast, these fractures are unstable under translational and rotational forces and thus require external stabilization that can be applied by a halo body vest. This brace fixates the head externally against the chest and thus prevents C-spine rotation along the ordinate axes.

In the thoracic and lumbar spine, the integrity of the posterior wall is a crucial indicator for stability of the fracture. The fracture can be addressed as bony stable if the vertebral body's posterior wall is intact. Functional mobilization featuring lordosing physiotherapy will be sufficient in compression injuries (Type A1), where the kyphosis of the end plates is less than 15°. In stable fractures with a greater degree of kyphosis, external stabilization is recommended after closed reduction is performed. Both the Boston Brace and a body cast will be sufficient in retaining the lordosis, if the principle of

Surgical Therapy

An absolute indication for operative intervention includes:

• Neurologic deficit
• High-grade instability
• Severe dislocation

- Failed closed reduction of spine dislocation
- Open spinal trauma

In patients with of neurologic deficit, especially with progressive deterioration, operative decompression must be performed on an emergency basis. Controversy exists as to whether an initially complete paraplegic patient will benefit from emergency decompression, because recovery is by definition impossible; however, we recommend initially treating these patients surgically, if instability, dislocation, or hematoma are detected, because it cannot be discerned in the early phase whether spinal shock mimics complete paraplegia.

Cervical Spine

In the upper C-spine, fractures of the odontoid process are most common. Operative treatment consists of an anterior screw fixation. In case of failed conservative treatment with formation of an odontoid process pseudarthrosis, posterior fixation may be indicated. The posterior atlanto-axial fusion technique was first described by Gallie, where sublaminar wiring is combined with a bone block that is attached onto the lamina. Magerl later described the transarticular screw fixation, where screws are passed through the articular mass between the course of the vertebral artery and the spinal canal. Harms recently described a technique in which polyaxial screws are driven into the lateral masses of both the atlas and the axis. This technique leaves the joint surfaces intact and thus is a motion-preserving technique when applied temporarily. In the lower C-spine, posterior fixation can be obtained by screw and rod systems, where the screws are either anchored in the lateral masses or transpedicularly (Fig. 7.4).

In general, anterior trauma (i.e., compression fracture of the vertebral body or discoligamentous lesion) is addressed by anterior approaches. Here the approach is chosen medial to the vascular sheath while the thyroid gland, larynx, and esophagus are retracted to the contralateral side. Stability is

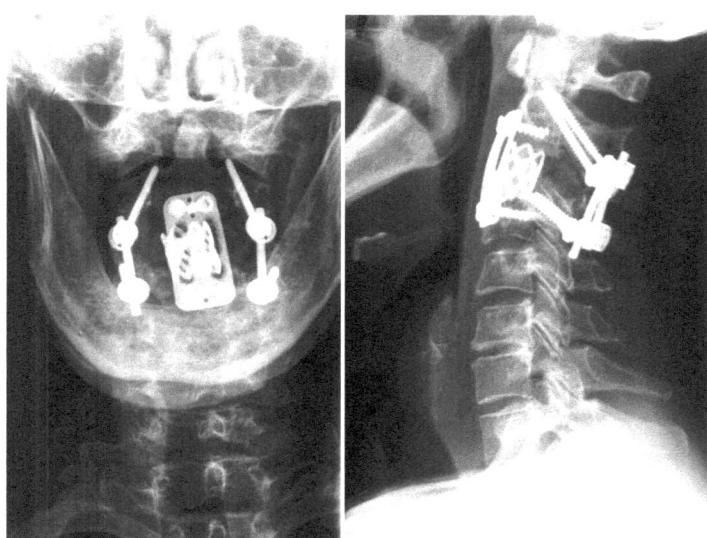

FIGURE 7.4. Stable instrumented fixation of a Type-C1 cervical fracture.

regained by insertion of a tricortical bone or a cage that is set under compression by anterior plating.

Thoracic and Lumbar Spine

During the preoperative planning, a decision must be made as to which approach is best suited to reduce, decompress, and stabilize the fracture. In addition, the patient's general condition must be evaluated. Operating time should be limited to the minimum in the polytraumatized patient in the early posttraumatic phase. In general, a posterior approach is recommended, through which reduction of the fracture and decompression can be achieved. In order to reconstruct a vertebral compression, stabilization of the anterior spine followed by insertion of tricortical bone or cage can be carried out via an anterior approach. In order to achieve the physiologic posterior tension, banding compression is applied to the posterior instrumentation. According to the individual situation of the patient, an initial anterior approach or a two-stage approach may be preferred.

The principles of surgical therapy are:

• Complete decompression of neural structures
• Reconstruction of a compression-stable anterior column
• Limitation of the fusion to the injured motion segment

Posterior procedures: The transpedicular screw anchorage introduced by Roy Camille and the further development of the internal fixator in which the screws are attached to rods in an angled stable construct have become the gold standard for the reduction and stabilization of spinal trauma. Because of the high pullout forces, there is no other fixation system available currently that offers similar stability. Depending on the surgeon's experience, the implant insertion may be aided by fluoroscopy or computerized navigation systems. A disadvantage of the open posterior approach is the resulting trauma to the paravertebral muscles. Thus, percutaneous internal fixators which offer both a minimal invasive insertion and reduction capacity are under clinical investigation currently; however, these instruments can only be used in cases where no open posterior decompression is necessary.

Anterior procedures: A stable reconstruction of the anterior column is necessary for all fractures of the thoracolumbar spine except some true distraction injuries (Type B2) of the thoracic spine.

Approaches: The thoracic spine may be approached via a thoracotomy either from the left or the right side depending on the extent of the fracture. The course of the approach via the intercostal space with opening of the pleura is quite painful in the postoperative course. This disadvantage led to the development of endoscopic techniques that may be applied if the reduction of the fracture was complete after the posterior instrumentation.

In the thoracolumbar junction, the diaphragm must be split in order to access the spine. Because both the abdominal and chest cavities are open, this approach is the most invasive access to the spine. The lower lumbar spine can be reached with a retroperitoneal or transperitoneal approach via lumbotomy or a transrectal incision. For access to L4 and L5, special care should be taken during the dissection of prevertebral large abdominal vessels.

In general, both tricortical bone crest and cages can be utilized as implants. The use of pressure stable cages, however, is recommended in the lumbar spine, because the size of the bone graft would result in remarkable donor site morbidity.

Complications

Because the spine features a unique proximity of osseus, neural, and vascular structures, there is a high potential for complications during the insertion of transpedicular screws. Decompression of the spinal canal might result in additional trauma of neural structures. In patients with SCI, the reduction maneuver with the internal fixator can worsen the neurologic situation. General medical complications include thrombosis, embolism, and pneumonia.

Postoperative Treatment and Prognosis

The advantage of the surgical treatment is the restoration of biomechanical stability. Thus patients can be mobilized en bloc immediately postoperatively. Depending on the quality of the bone stock and the resulting stability of the instrumentation, an external brace with a three-point support is prescribed for a period of 12 weeks. Implant removal of the posterior instrumentation may be carried out after 6 months.

Full physical activity is regained after 6 months depending on the bony fusion as evaluated radiologically. Accelerated degeneration of the adjacent segments might occur in the long term as reported as a late sequel of fusion surgery. The long-term prognosis of paraplegic patients often depends on the quality of the rehabilitation. Modern comprehensive care is a multidisciplinary approach comprising orthopedic surgeons, neurologists, physiotherapists, occupational therapists, and nursing specialists.

Evidence-Based Medicine

The treatment of spinal injuries has changed over the past decades. Due to the clinical implementation of Advanced Trauma Life Support (ATLS), spinal trauma is treated adequately in the early stages of trauma care. With the introduction of newer surgical techniques (anterior column spacers, posterior screw rod systems), great advances have been achieved in stable instrumentation of the injured spine for immediate postoperative mobilization. Criticism has been given, however, that many technical and material advances were adopted frequently without scientific evidence. Evidence-based medicine (EBM) not only assesses objective measures but also takes patient-focused outcomes such as self-reported questionnaires into account.

Controversy persists about the value of high-dose administration of corticosteroids. Since the publication of the National Acute Spinal Cord Injury Study (NASCIS-II), there has been an increase in the administration of methylprednisolone in patients with spinal cord trauma. Recent studies have not proven unequivocally better results in the final assessment of patients who received corticosteroids. More research is needed in order to evaluate precisely which kind of SCI benefits from the anti-inflammatory medication.

Also it is not clear that early surgical decompression leads to more favorable results in patients with SCI. While animal studies show an excellent recovery of neural function after immediate decompression, it has been difficult to acquire evidence in the clinical scenario. Currently, there is a prospective observational study underway (Surgical Treatment of

Acute Spinal Cord Injury Study—STASCIS) in order to provide better evidence toward optimal timing of surgical intervention. In contrast, there seems to be a consensus that early surgical stabilization is indicated in neurologically intact patients for reduction of complications resulting from immobilization.

Selected Readings

Anderson LD, D'Alonzo RT (1974) Fractures of the odontoid process of the axis. J Bone J Surg 56A:663

Bracken MB, Shepard MJ, Collins WF, et al. (1990) A randomized controlled trial of methyl-prednisolone or naloxone in the treatment of acute spinal cord injury. N Engl J Med 322:1406

Magerl F, Aebi M, Gertzbein SD, et al. (1994) A comprehensive classification of thoracic and lumbar injuries. Eur Spine J 3:184

Pickett GE, Campos-Benitez M, Keller JL, Dugall N (2006) Epidemiology of traumatic spinal cord injury in Canada. Spine 31:799

Roy-Camille R, Saillant G, Berteaux D, Marie-Anne S (1979) Early management of spinal injuries. In: McKibbin B (ed) Recent advances in orthopaedics 3. Churchill Livingstone, Edinburgh, pp 57–87

Whitesides TE Jr (1977) Traumatic kyphosis of the thoracolumbar spine. Clin Orthop 128:78

8
Abdominal Compartment Syndrome

Hanns-Peter Knaebel

Pearls and Pitfalls

- Abdominal compartment syndrome (ACS) is a life-threatening disease.
- Primary, secondary, and tertiary ACS are being recognized recently.
- Primary ACS is associated with abdominal trauma.
- Secondary ACS is a condition caused mostly by ischemia and reperfusion.
- Tertiary ACS is the condition of persistent intra-abdominal hypertension.
- Clinical diagnosis and imaging of ACS is difficult. Early diagnosis is crucial.
- The gold standard of diagnosis remains the measurement of intra-abdominal pressure.
- The critical value of abdominal pressure is between 15 and 20 mmHg.
- Conservative options are extremely important, but conservative treatment of intra abdominal pressures >25 mmHg is usually not effective.
- Decompressive laparotomy is the ultimate therapeutic option to reduce mortality.

K.I. Bland et al. (eds.), *Trauma Surgery*,
DOI 10.1007/978-1-84996-375-6_8,
© Springer-Verlag London Limited 2011

Introduction

For many years, abdominal compartment syndrome (ACS) seemed like a forgotten entity or at least a medical condition that physicians and especially surgeons refrained from discussing. In recent years, there has been a substantial increase in knowledge and interest relating to ACS. This chapter will outline some recent developments.

Definitions

In December 2004, the World Congress on the Abdominal Compartment Syndrome was held, with 170 leaders from around the world setting the stage for future understanding of this complex physiologic phenomenon and developing common definitions to facilitate concise academic exchange.

Intra-Abdominal Pressure

Intra-abdominal pressure (IAP) is the pressure within the abdominal cavity. IAP varies with respiration. Normal IAP is approximately 5 mmHg, but it can be increased non-pathologically in obese patients. IAP should be expressed in mmHg (1 mmHg = 1.36 cm H_2O) and measured at end-expiration with the patient in the supine position; abdominal muscle contractions should be absent. The transducer should be zeroed at the level of the midaxillary line. The most accurate method for direct, invasive IAP measurement is direct needle puncture and transduction of the pressure within the abdominal cavity (e.g., during peritoneal dialysis or laparoscopy), but the gold standard for intermittent, indirect, non-invasive IAP measurement is transduction of the pressure within the bladder. The reference method for continuous indirect IAP measurement is a balloon-tipped catheter in the stomach or a continuous bladder irrigation method. The relevant value to be calculated is the abdominal perfusion pressure = mean arterial pressure – IAP.

Intra-Abdominal Hypertension

Intra-abdominal hypertension (IAH) is defined by either one or both of the following: (1) an IAP of 12 mmHg or greater, recorded by a minimum of three standardized measurements conducted 4–6 h apart; (2) an abdominal perfusion pressure of 60 mmHg or less, recorded by a minimum of two standardized measurements conducted 1–6 h apart.

Abdominal Compartment Syndrome

Abdominal compartment syndrome is defined as the presence of an IAP of 20 mmHg or greater with or without abdominal perfusion pressure below 50 mmHg, recorded by a minimum of three standardized measurements conducted 1–6 h apart and single or multiple organ system failure that was not present previously. In contrast to IAH, ACS should not be graded, because it is an all-or-nothing phenomenon leading to immediate therapeutic consequences. IAH is graded as shown in Table 8.1.

TABLE 8.1. Proposed grading system for abdominal compartment syndrome based on intra-abdominal pressure.

Grade	IAP (mmHg)	Associated signs	Treatment
I	10–15	No signs of ACS	Maintain normovolemia
II	16–25	May have increased PAWP* and oliguria	Hypervolemic resuscitation may be employed but could have drawbacks
III	26–35	Anuria, decreased cardiac output, raised PAWP	Consider abdominal decompression
IV	>35	Anuria, decreased cardiac output, raised PAWP	Abdominal decompression and re-exploration (cave tertiary ACS: avoid primary abdominal wall closure)

*PAWP: pulmonary artery wedge pressure.

Prevalence of Intra-Abdominal Hypertension and Abdominal Compartment Syndrome

The prevalence of IAH in the literature is variable, depending on the threshold used to define IAH and the population studied. A recent multi-center group performed a prospective study of IAH in a mixed intensive care unit (ICU) population. In this study, 265 consecutive patients (mean Acute Physiology and Chronic Health Evaluation II (APACHE II) score 17.4) admitted for more than 24 h in one of the 14 participating ICUs were monitored until death, until hospital discharge, or for a maximum of 28 days. Medical patients accounted for 47% of all study patients, whereas elective surgery, emergency surgery, and trauma patients accounted for 28%, 17%, and 9%, respectively. IAH was present when the mean value of the two daily IAP measurements was greater than 12 mmHg. ACS was diagnosed when an IAP above 20 mmHg was associated with at least one organ failure.

On admission, 32% of the population had IAH, and 4% had ACS. Importantly, unlike the occurrence of IAH at day 1, the occurrence of IAH during ICU stay was an independent predictor of mortality. Independent predictors of IAH at day 1 were liver dysfunction, abdominal surgery, fluid resuscitation with more than 3,500 ml during the 24 h before inclusion, and ileus. Previously, we showed that grade 2 IAH (16–20 mmHg) occurs in more than 30% of patients undergoing emergency surgery. Despite increasing reporting of ACS and IAH in the literature, the importance of IAH is often ignored.

Thus, it needs to be noted that the true prevalence of the disease as well as the predisposing risk factors are not completely known and understood (see Table 8.2). Regardless of the uncertainties, it is extremely important to appreciate the severity of the disease because mortality ranges from 29% to 100%.

TABLE 8.2. Risk factors, etiology and definitions of abdominal compartment syndrome (ACS).

Primary ACS	Secondary ACS	Tertiary ACS
Blunt or penetrating abdominal trauma with hemorrhage	Extensive fluid resuscitation following major trauma	Recurrent or persistent ACS following prophylactic or therapeutic surgical or medical treatment of ACS (e.g., persistence after decompressive laparotomy, new ACS after definite abdominal wall closure)
Abdomino-pelvic trauma/injury and retroperitoneal hemorrhage	Forced abdominal wall closure (AWC) following peritonitis, ileus or intra-abdominal abscess	
Ruptured aortic aneurysm	Laparoscopy and pneumoperitoneum	
Ascites formation due to liver cirrhosis, malignoma or pregnancy	Abdominal packing following hemorrhage	
Any other condition that requires early surgical or angio-radiologic intervention (e.g., secondary peritonitis)	Any other condition not originating from an abdominal disease (e.g., sepsis or major burns)	

New Trends in Monitoring Intra-Abdominal Pressure Measurement

There have been significant developments in IAP monitoring. Balogh et al. validated prospectively the technique of continuous IAP monitoring and showed that this new method has almost a perfect agreement with the reference standard of Kron et al. of intermittent measurements of intra-vesical IAP. There are many obvious advantages of the described continuous IAP monitoring. First, it does not require a major change in the present practice apart from the use of three-way urinary catheters. This method abandons the cumbersome steps of draining, clamping of the catheter, and filling with 50 ml of normal saline. The monitoring is continuous and does not interfere with the urinary flow through the drainage port of the catheter. Continuous IAP monitoring is less labor intensive and time consuming compared with the standard intermittent measuring technique. These factors will lead to a greater acceptance of IAP monitoring in patients at risk. The indications for monitoring IAP are presented in Table 8.3.

Continuous IAP measurement has several potential advantages. Increasingly, Signal Interpretation and Monitoring will become a more powerful tool for physiologic monitoring.

TABLE 8.3. Indications for monitoring of intra-abdominal pressure (IAP).

Indication
Postoperative patients after extensive abdominal surgery
Patients with open or blunt abdominal trauma
Mechanically ventilated ICU patients with other organ dysfunction as assessed by daily Sequential Organ Failure
Assessment score (SOFA score)
Patients with a distended abdomen and signs and symptoms consistent with abdominal compartment syndrome: oliguria, hypoxia, hypotension, unexplained acidosis, mesenteric ischemia, elevated ventilating pressure, elevated intracranial pressure

Continuous measurement of the IAP facilitates monitoring the abdominal perfusion pressure both intermittently and continuously.

Pathophysiology

Intra-abdominal pressure is determined primarily by the volume of the viscera and the intra-compartmental fluid load. The pressure-volume curve of the abdominal cavity has been studied in animals. Post-mortem evaluation of human pressure-volume curves may not be reliable because of the post-mortem loss of abdominal wall compliance. In general, the abdominal cavity has a great tolerance to fluctuating volumes, with little increase in IAP. The compliance of the abdominal cavity can be seen at laparoscopy, wherein it is possible to instill as much as 5 l of CO_2 into the peritoneal cavity without exerting any marked influence on IAP. In a previous evaluation of IAP during laparoscopy, we found that the mean volume of gas required to generate a pressure of 20 mmHg was 8.8 ± 4.3 l. Adaptation can occur over time, and this is seen clinically in patients with ascites, large ovarian tumors, and, of course, pregnancy. Chronic ACS occurs in some morbidly obese patients with significantly increased IAP predisposing to chronic venous stasis, urinary incontinence, incisional hernia, and intracranial hypertension. Definitions and etiology of ACS is shown in Table 8.2.

Effect of Increased Intra-Abdominal Pressure on Individual Organ Function

Whereas intra-abdominal hypertension has a global affect on the body, increasing intraabdominal pressure leading to ACS tends to affect one system first, usually the renal or gastrointestinal system. The selective affects of IAH will be discussed in the following section.

Renal

Renal dysfunction in association with increased IAP has been recognized for more than 100 years, but only recently have its effects on large series of patients been reported. In 1945 in a study of 17 volunteers, there was a reduction in renal plasma flow and glomerular filtration rate in association with increased IAP. In an animal experiment, as IAP increased from 0 to 20 mmHg in dogs, the glomerular filtration rate decreased by 25%. At 40 mmHg, the dogs were resuscitated, and their cardiac output returned to normal; however their glomerular filtration rate and renal blood flow did not improve, indicating a local effect on renal blood flow. The situation in seriously ill patients may, however, be different, and the exact cause of renal dysfunction in the ICU is not clear because of the complexity of critical illness.

The most likely direct effect of increased IAP is an increase in the renal vascular resistance, combined with a moderate resultant decrease in cardiac output. Pressure on the ureter can be excluded as a cause, because investigators placing ureteric stents observed no improvement in renal function and urinary excretion. Other factors contributing to renal dysfunction may include humeral factors and intraparenchymal renal pressures. The concept of renal decapsulation, on the basis of increased intrarenal pressure, was popular some decades ago but now is practiced rarely because it is of no proven benefit.

The absolute value of IAP required to cause renal impairment has not been established. Some authors have suggested that 10–15 mmHg is a critical cut-off value. Maintaining adequate cardiovascular filling pressures in the presence of increased IAP also seems to be of importance.

Cardiovascular

Increased IAP decreases cardiac output as well as increasing central venous pressure, systemic vascular resistance, pulmonary artery pressure, and pulmonary artery wedge pressure. It should be kept in mind that because of the associated increase in intra-pleural pressure, some of the increases in central venous pressure may not reflect the intravascular volume and may be misleading when the patient's volume status is assessed. Cardiac output is affected mainly by a decrease in stroke volume secondary to a decrease in preload and an increase in afterload which is further aggravated by hypovolemia. Paradoxically, in the presence of hypovolemia, an increase in IAP can be associated temporarily with an increase in cardiac output. The normal left atrial/right atrial pressure gradient may be reversed during increased IAP. Venous stasis occurs in the legs of patients with abdominal pressures above 12 mmHg. In addition, studies in patients undergoing laparoscopic cholecystectomy show up to a fourfold increase in renin and aldosterone levels.

Respiration

Animal as well as human experiments have demonstrated that IAP exerts a marked effect on pulmonary function. In conjunction with increased IAP, there is diaphragmatic stenting, exerting a restrictive effect on the lungs with a resultant decrease in ventilation and lung compliance, an increase in airway pressures, and a reduction in tidal volumes. These changes can be seen occasionally during laparoscopy, where lung compliance has been shown to decrease once the IAP exceeds 16 mmHg. Respiratory changes related to increased IAP are aggravated by increased obesity and other physiologic conditions such as severe hemorrhage. There is also some adverse effect on the efficiency of gas exchange. Often patients with increased IAP are acidotic, and whereas this acidosis may initially be metabolic in origin, the effect of increased IAP adds a component complicating respiration.

In critically ill patients receiving ventilation, the effect on the respiratory system can be clinically important, resulting in decreased lung volumes, impaired gas exchange, and high ventilatory pressures. Hypercarbia can occur, and the resulting acidosis can be exacerbated by simultaneous cardiovascular depression as a result of increased IAP. The effects of increased IAP on the respiratory system in the ICU can sometimes be life-threatening, and require urgent abdominal decompression (see Figs. 8.1 and 8.2). In patients with true ACS undergoing abdominal decompression, there is a remarkable change in intra-operative vital signs. Fortunately, these patients represent the minority rather than a majority of patients with increased IAP and ACS. Frankly, patients should never be allowed to get to this stage. Monitoring of vital signs and acid-base status is vital in this patient population.

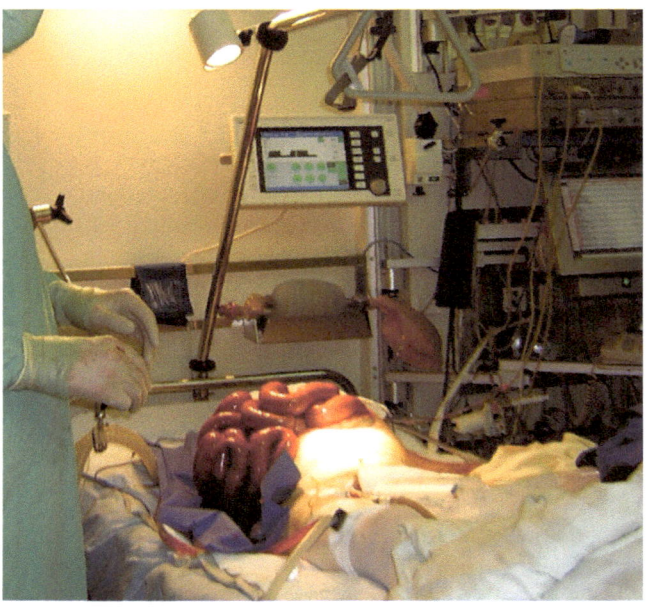

FIGURE 8.1. ACS due to SIRS following total pancreatectomy immediately after emergency decompressive laparotomy on the surgical ICU. Due to extremely increased ventilation pressures, the patient could not be transported to the operating room. The impaired perfusion of the small bowel is striking.

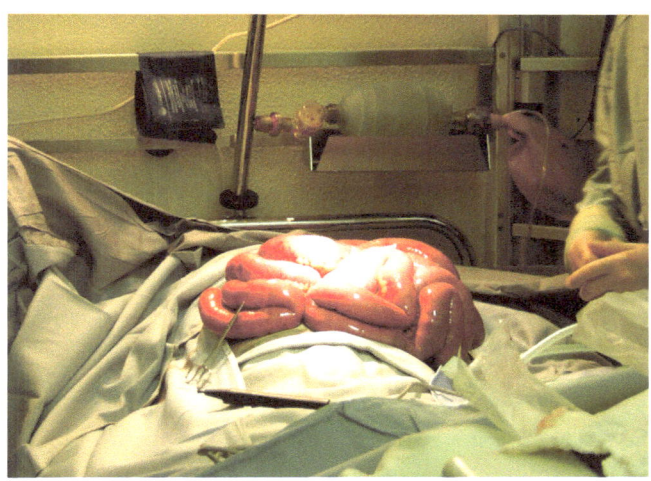

FIGURE 8.2. Same patient as in Fig. 8.1, 15 min after laparotomy. The small bowel is distended grossly due a paralytic ileus, however the perfusion recovered. Next steps were decompression of the small bowel via intraluminal suction and vacuum-assisted wound closure to avoid tertiary ACS.

Visceral Perfusion

Interest in visceral perfusion has increased with the popularization of gastric tonometry, and there is an association between IAP and visceral perfusion as measured by gastric pH (intestinal pH = pHi – Value). This observation was confirmed in 18 patients undergoing laparoscopy in whom a reduction of 15–54% in blood flow occurred in the duodenum and stomach, respectively, at an IAP of 15 mmHg. Animal studies suggest that reduction in visceral perfusion is selective, affecting intestinal blood flow before adrenal blood flow. In a study of 73 post-laparotomy patients, IAP and pHi were associated strongly, suggesting that early decreases in visceral perfusion are related to levels of IAP as low as 15 mmHg. Increasing IAP may result in visceral hypoperfusion and subsequently in secondary bacterial translocation as well as affecting wound healing.

Both abnormal pHi and IAP predicted the same adverse outcome with increased risk of hypotension, intra-abdominal sepsis, renal impairment, need for re-laparotomy, and fatal outcome. It is important to measure IAP to increase awareness of its potential adverse effects on the gut. The indications for IAP monitoring are shown in Table 8.3.

Conservative Treatment Options

The precise management of IAP remains somewhat clouded by many published anecdotal reports and uncontrolled case series. Aggressive, non-operative intensive care support is critical to prevent the establishment of and the complications of ACS.

This approach involves careful monitoring of the cardiorespiratory system and aggressive intravascular fluid replacement, especially if this is associated with hemorrhage. In contrast, excessive fluid resuscitation will add to the problem. Simple measures such as naso-gastric decompression are mandatory. In Table 8.4 some of the possible non-surgical

TABLE 8.4. Non-surgical therapeutic options for the treatment of intra-abdominal hypertension (IAH) and for the prevention of abdominal compartment syndrome (ACS).

Conservative therapy
Paracentesis
Naso-gastric tubes with gastric suctioning
Gastricprokinetics (metoclopramide, erythromycin, etc.)
Rectal enemas and suctioning
Colonicprokinetics (prostigmine)
Furosemide either alone or in combination with human albumin 20%
Continuous venovenous hemo(dia)filtration with aggressive ultrafiltration
Continuous negative abdominal pressure
Sedation and muscle relaxation
Upright (sitting) body positioning (pilot seat)

options are shown which all have the intention of preventing the full clinical symptoms of ACS.

Surgical Management

As yet, there are few guidelines for when surgical decompression is required in the presence of increased IAP. Some studies have stated that abdominal decompression is the only treatment and that it should be performed early to prevent ACS. This is an overstatement not supported by level 1 evidence.

The accepted indications for abdominal decompression are related to correcting pathophysiologic abnormalities as much as achieving a precise and optimum IAP. If gas exchange is increasingly compromised with collapse of the lung bases or ventilatory pressures are increasing, abdominal decompression should be considered strongly. Similarly, if cardiovascular or renal function is compromised and increased IAP is suspected, then decompression should be considered early. Unfortunately, visceral hypoperfusion is very difficult to predict apart from gastric tonometry, and guidelines for operative intervention would have to rely on levels of IAP that have been shown to correlate with visceral ischemia.

The approaches to abdominal decompression also vary. Temporary abdominal closure (TAC) has been popularized as a mechanism to avoid many of the consequences of increased IAP. The theoretic benefits of abdominal decompression and TAC are therefore attractive, and some authors have advocated the prophylactic use of TAC to decrease post-operative complications and facilitate planned re-laparotomy (see Fig. 8.3); however, this approach may be hard to justify until a subgroup of high-risk patients can be identified more accurately. Burch et al. have stated that abdominal decompression can reverse the sequelae of the ACS. IAP levels have been advocated as a guide to closure of the abdominal wall, especially in children, but the existing literature currently has few prospective studies. Wittman et al. in two separate studies in 1990 and 1994 evaluated prospectively the outcomes in 157 and 95 patients, respectively. A multi-institutional study of 95

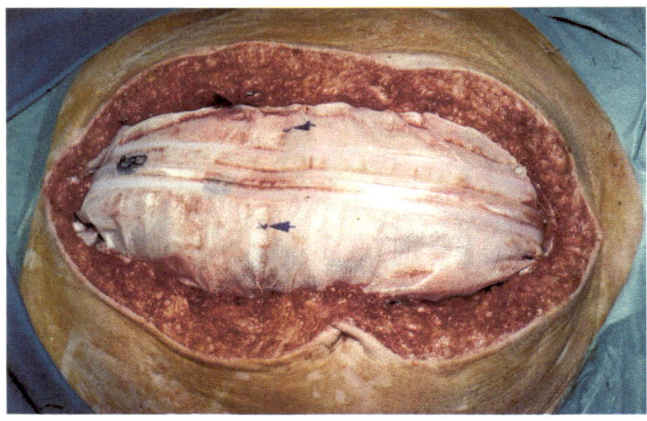

FIGURE 8.3. Temporary abdominal wound closure ("zipper") after necrotizing pancreatitis and ACS to facilitate repeated laparotomy and to avoid tertiary ACS.

patients concluded that a staged approach to abdominal closure with TAC was superior to conventional techniques for dealing with intra-abdominal sepsis. Rock-hard evidence, however, is still missing.

The common indications for performing TAC include the following: abdominal decompression both prophylactic and therapeutic; to facilitate re-exploration in abdominal sepsis; and inability to close the abdomen. One must remember, however, that the open abdomen is not without its morbidity, needs intensive wound care and attention, and should be re-constructed whenever possible and feasible (see Fig. 8.4).

Conclusion

Increasingly, intra-abdominal hypertension (IAH) and abdominal compartment syndrome (ACS) are being recognized and diagnosed and are no longer considered a curiosity or a "forgotten entity." The challenge lies not in identifying

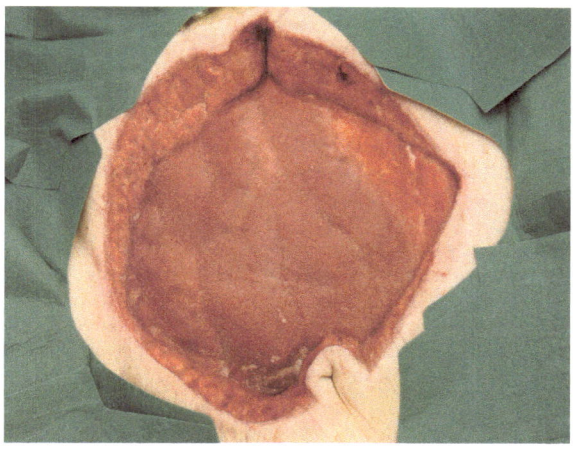

FIGURE 8.4. Same patient as in Figs. 8.1 and 8.2 after vacuum-assisted wound conditioning prior to plastic reconstruction of the abdominal wall. The small bowel is covered nicely with granulation tissue.

predictors of ACS but in optimizing conservative, early-onset treatment as well the operative treatment options, including identifying when and in whom abdominal decompression is necessary. Thus, it seems reasonable that the newly formed Society of the Abdominal Compartment Syndrome will act as a portal for discussion, clinical trials, and research to enhance understanding and optimize patient care.

Selected Readings

Balogh Z, Moore FA (2005) Intra-abdominal hypertension: not just a surgical critical care curiosity. Crit Care Med 33:447–449

Balogh Z, McKinley BA, Cocanour CS, et al. (2003) Supra-normal trauma resuscitation causes more cases of abdominal compartment syndrome. Arch Surg 138:637–642; discussion 642–633

Balogh Z, Jones F, D'Amours S, et al. (2004) Continuous intra-abdominal pressure measurement technique. Am J Surg 188:679–684

Burch J, Moore E, Moore F, Franciose R (1996) The abdominal compartment syndrome. Surg Clin North Am 76:833–842

Caldwell CB, Ricotta JJ (1987) Changes in visceral blood flow with elevated intra-abdominal pressure. J Surg Res 43:14–20

Harman KP, Kron IL, McLachlan DH (1982) Elevated intra-abdominal pressure and renal function. Ann Surg 196:594–597

Kron IL, Harman PK, Nolan SP (1984) The measurement of intraabdominal pressure as a criterion for abdominal re-exploration. Ann Surg 196:594–597

Malbrain ML (2004) Different techniques to measure intraabdominal pressure (IAP): time for a critical reappraisal. Intensive Care Med 30:357–371

Malbrain ML, Chiumello D, Pelosi P, et al. (2005) Incidence and prognosis of intraabdominal hypertension in a mixed population of critically ill patients: a multiple-center epidemiological study. Crit Care Med 33:315–322

Pusajo J, Bumaschny E, Agurrola A, et al. (1994) Postoperative intra-abdominal pressure: its relation to splanchnic perfusion, sepsis, multiple organ failure and surgical intervention. Intensive Crit Care Digest 13:2–7

World Society of the Abdominal Compartment Syndrome. www.wsacs.org

9
Neurologic Physiology: The Brain and Its Response to Injury

Mamerhi O. Okor and James M. Markert

Pearls and Pitfalls

- Early clinical recognition and radiographic diagnosis are key initial steps in the management of head injury.
- Once a surgical lesion has been ruled out in a severely head-injured patient, aggressive medical management should be instituted. Medical management primarily constitutes supportive therapy aimed at preventing secondary insults to the brain, which should include the detection and treatment of raised intracranial pressure (ICP).
- In the event that first-line therapy for the management of elevated ICPs is unsuccessful, "second-tier" therapy may be cautiously applied.
- Lack of an aggressive initial approach to the head-injured patient can lead to an exacerbation of the initial injury due to potentially avoidable secondary injury – an inadequate resuscitation can lead to superimposed hypoxic or ischemic injury, and delayed institution of measures to combat increased ICP can result in increases in local tissue pressures and local ischemia, or even avoidable herniation syndromes.
- A poor neurologic exam in the setting of an initially normal-appearing computed tomography (CT) scan may be due to toxic/metabolic issues, but also can be a result of a hypoxic injury or diffuse axonal injury (DAI).

K.I. Bland et al. (eds.), *Trauma Surgery*,
DOI 10.1007/978-1-84996-375-6_9,
© Springer-Verlag London Limited 2011

- An early accurate neurologic assessment can prevent the clinician from delaying the diagnosis of an intracranial mass lesion that may require immediate operative intervention, particularly if a unilateral fixed and dilated pupil is present, or a patient has a marked hemiparesis.
- Patients in whom such an exam is not possible due to pharmacologic paralysis before such an assessment can be undertaken, require an urgent head CT to avoid missing such a diagnosis.
- Overuse of hyperventilation (prolonged periods of $PaCO_2$ of 25 mmHg or less) can result in rebound intracranial hypertension; $PaCO_2$ should generally be kept in the 30–35 mmHg range. Serum osmolarity should be maintained below 310–320 to minimize the risk of renal injury in the setting of prolonged mannitol administration, and switching to hyperosmolar saline use in these patients can decrease this risk.
- Avoidable use of pharmacologic paralysis can lead to sepsis, pneumonia, and increased ICU stays.

Classification of Brain Injury

Closed head injury can be classified based on severity (mild, moderate, or severe) which is determined largely by Glasgow Coma Scale scoring; mechanism (missile or blunt); and pathology (primary or secondary). A prompt and thorough initial neurologic assessment is crucial in determining the nature of a patient's injury and instituting the appropriate treatment protocol.

Missile Injuries

Missile injuries can be classified as depressed, penetrating, or perforating. In *depressed injuries*, the missile fails to penetrate the skull but produces a depressed skull fracture and/or causes a contusional injury to the underlying brain. Brain damage is therefore focal, and consciousness is rarely altered for long. In *penetrating injuries*, the missile enters the cranial cavity but does not leave it. If the object is small and sharp, and penetration is limited, little direct injury to the skull and brain may occur. The damage is focal, and the patient seldom loses consciousness. However, the missile may penetrate deeply enough to damage vital structures. Penetration through multiple lobes, both hemispheres, the ventricular system, or posterior fossa involvement by the missile will all produce more extensive damage. Even simple penetrating head injuries may allow infection, meningitis, or cerebral abscesses to develop. In a penetrating injury, the missile (usually a bullet) passes and exits the brain but does not leave the skull, resulting in a penetrating brain wound. If the bullet exits the head, the injury is called a *perforating head injury*. The exit wound in the skull is characteristically larger than the entry wound. Low-velocity missiles rarely exit the skull, although they often produce multiple destructive tracts through the brain in which there may be bone fragments, soft tissues, and clothing. Although a high-velocity bullet may pass through the head without causing impairment of consciousness, brain damage in these circumstances tend to be severe and extensive, likely due to the shockwaves generated by the missile. Any missile injury can result in the formation of a hematoma, which can further complicate injury management and patient outcome.

Blunt Injuries

Blunt injuries frequently result in scalp lacerations, skull fractures, contusions, subdural hematomas (SDHs), epidural hematomas (EDHs), and axonal shear injuries. *Scalp lacerations* can be of considerable importance as sources of blood loss and indications of the site of injury. If there is an associated depressed skull fracture, scalp lacerations represent a potential avenue for intracranial infection.

Skull fractures may involve the cranial vault or skull base and may be classified as linear or depressed. The frequency of skull fractures appears to correlate with the severity of head injury.

Patients with a fracture have a much higher incidence of intracranial hematoma than patients without a fracture. A depressed skull fracture is considered to be compound if an associated scalp laceration extending through the pericranium is present, and penetrating if a dural laceration exists. Depressed fractures are more likely to provide potential routes for intracranial infections than linear fractures, and are associated with an increased incidence of post-traumatic epilepsy. Skull base fractures may also be complicated by intracranial infections, as organisms may spread from the air sinuses or the middle ear, especially in the setting of an undiagnosed or untreated cerebrospinal fluid (CSF) fistula (CSF rhinorrhea or otorrhea).

Intracranial hemorrhage is a common complication of head injury and is the most common cause of clinical deterioration and death in patients who experienced a lucid interval after injury. Intracranial injury may be subdivided into extra-axial hematomas, which include EDHs, SDHs, subarachnoid hemorrhages, and intracerebral hematomas which arise within the parenchyma of the brain. Although intracranial hematomas can be identified on initial CT evaluation, the severity of its clinical manifestations along with the potential for delayed neurologic deterioration are due in large part to the time it takes for the hematoma to attain a size sufficient to cause brain distortion and herniation, as well as the development of associated edema. Expanding hematomas should be distinguished from delayed hematomas, which are described as lesions that occur more than 24 h after the time of injury that are not evident on initial imaging studies.

Most intracranial hematomas develop within the first 48 h after injury, but SDHs may also be subacute (2–14 days after injury) or chronic (more than 14 days after injury).

Epidural hematomas or EDHs (Fig. 9.1) often result from hemorrhage from a meningeal artery, most often a branch of the middle meningeal artery, and are associated with overlying skull fractures in 90% of adult patients. The incidence of skull fractures is lower in children with EDHs. EDHs occur most often in the temporal region but 25% occur elsewhere, such as in the frontal and parietal regions or within the posterior fossa, where they may occur as a result of venous sinus injury.

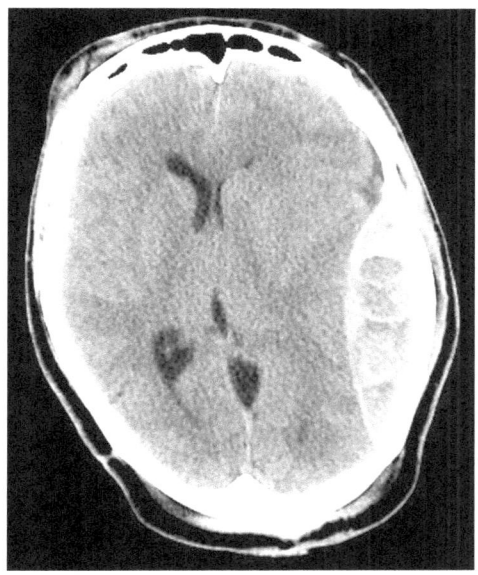

FIGURE 9.1. Epidural hematoma. Note the lentiform nature and the significant mass effect on the ventricular system, with left to right shift. Most of these lesions arise from damage to the middle meningeal artery or other dural vessels, and are often associated with skull fractures.

Occasionally, these hematomas are multiple. As the hematoma enlarges, it strips the dural from the skull, forming an elliptical mass that is limited by the dural investment into the calvarial sutures. In patients who experience a lucid interval, there is often little evidence of other types of brain injury. If however, the patient has been in a coma from the time of the original injury, other types of brain injury are likely to be present. Isolated EDHs of <30 ml in volume infrequently cause an alteration in the level of consciousness or a focal neurologic deficit.

Subdural hematomas or SDHs (Fig. 9.2) are brought on by the rupture of the bridging veins that connect cortical veins to dural venous sinuses or from a laceration in a cortical artery. Subdural veins are sensitive to the rate at which they are

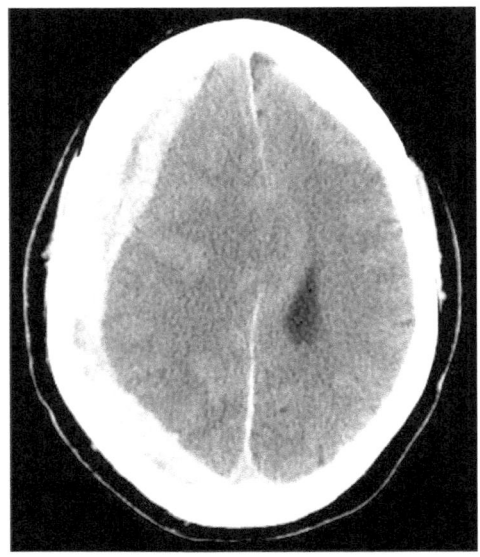

FIGURE 9.2. Subdural hematoma (SDH). Note the convex shape of the lesion. SDHs are usually associated with acute underlying brain injury and generally have a worse prognosis than epidural hematomas (EDHs).

deformed by acceleration (strain-sensitive). The general mobidity and mortality rates are greater for subdural hematomas than for EDHs because of the higher incidence of concurrent brain damage. SDHs are classified by their appearance, classically on CT imaging, as follows: acute when the hematoma is composed of clotted blood that appears hyperdense to brain tissue on noncontrast head CT; subacute when composed of a mixture of clotted and fluid blood that appears isodense to brain tissue; or chronic when composed purely of liquefied blood and proteins mixed with CSF that appears hypodense to brain tissue. The clotted blood remains for at least 48 h and sometimes several days. The transition to a more fluid blood is largely due to the action of fibrinolytic enzymes that dissolve the clot. These enzymes start this dissolution within 72–96 h after clot formation. After about 3 weeks, no clot remains. In about 25% of patients who undergo evacuation of an acute SDH, acute brain edema occurs in the hemisphere underlying the clot and portends a poor prognosis.

Cerebral contusions have long since been considered the hallmark of head injury. Contusions occur characteristically in the frontal and temporal poles and on the inferior surfaces of the frontal and temporal lobes where the brain tissue comes in contact with the protuberances at the skull base. In early stages, they are hemorrhagic and swollen, but with time they evolve into shrunken gliotic scars. Because the damage ful recovery from head injury, provided that they do not develop complications leading to other types of brain damage and that they do not sustain diffuse axonal injury (DAI) at the time of original injury. Contusions can be further subdivided into fracture contusions, coup contusions, contra-coup contusions, and herniation contusions. Fracture contusions occur at the site of a fracture and are particularly severe in the frontal lobe. Coup contusions occur at the site of injury in the absence of a fracture. Contra-coup contusions in the brain occur diametrically opposed to the point of injury as a result of brain movement within the calvarium. Herniation contusions occur when the medial parts of the temporal lobes are impacted against the edge of the tentorium, or the cerebellar tonsils are impacted against the foramen magnum at the site of the injury.

Intracerebral hematomas (Fig. 9.3) are found in approximately 15% of all patients who sustain fatal head injuries. These hematomas may be single or multiple, and occur primarily in the frontal and temporal regions. They most likely result from a direct rupture of intrinsic cerebral blood vessel in relation to contusions at the time of injury.

Diffuse axonal injury, or DAI, occurs when the head and brain are subject to severe rotational forces, and is characterized by the shearing of nerve fibers at the moment of injury. The clinical presentation of DAI remains varied. Patients may present with brief periods of altered consciousness or may

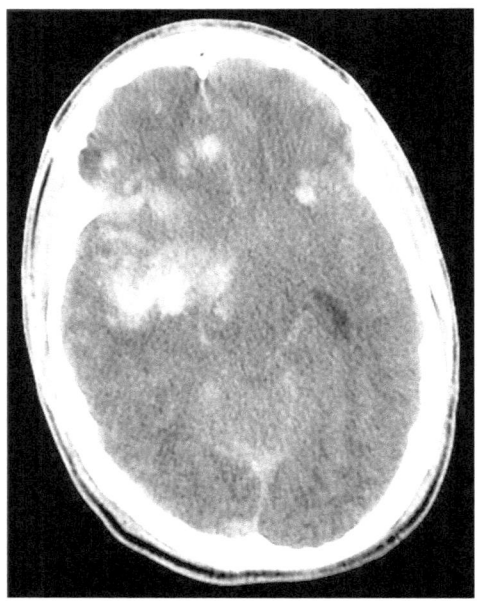

FIGURE 9.3. Multiple intraparenchymal hematomas. These lesions arise within the parenchyma of the brain itself and indicate a significant injury to the brain itself. They can produce mass effect and also may evolve over the days post-injury to produce edema, which may produce increases in ICP if the hematoma is not evacuated surgically.

remain in a coma for extended periods of time. In severe cases, patients with DAI are left in a persistent vegetative state or may expire depending on the severity of concurrent secondary injury. Patients with DAI have a statistically lower incidence of lucid intervals, skull fractures, cerebral contusions, intracerebral hematomas, and evidence of elevated intracranial pressures (ICPs). In the absence of magnetic resonance imaging (MRI) or characteristic CT findings, the diagnosis of DAI is largely exclusionary, encompassing a spectrum of patients with severe closed head injury and a paucity of findings on noncontrast head CT. In its most severe form, DAI is characterized by focal lesions in the corpus callosum, focal lesions in the dorsolateral aspect of the rostral brainstem, and evidence of diffuse injury to axons. These focal lesions may be evident as petechial hemorrhages on a noncontrast CT scan. Since the advent of the MRI with its high sensitivity for parenchymal injury, the definition of DAI has been expanded to include patients with nonhemorrhagic areas of T2 signal within the white matter or at the gray–white junction.

Secondary Brain Injury

An increase in the volume of all or part of the brain is common in patients who sustain severe blunt head injury. The resultant edema may be severe enough to raise the ICP and cause death from brain shift, herniation, and secondary damage to the brainstem. The brain swelling is largely due to an increase in cerebral blood volume (congestive brain swelling) or water content of the brain tissue (cerebral edema). Brain swelling can be classified into three types: swelling adjacent to contusions, diffuse swelling of one cerebral hemisphere, and diffuse swelling of both cerebral hemispheres.

Swelling of the brain adjacent to contusions is common and is due to physical disruption of the tissue with damage to the blood brain barrier and loss of normal physiologic autoregulation of arterioles. Water and electrolytes leak into the brain tissue and spread into the adjacent white matter.

Diffuse swelling of one cerebral hemisphere is most often seen in association with an ipsilateral acute SDH. When the hematoma is evacuated, the brain simply expands to fill the space created. This is attributed to engorgement of a nonreactive vascular bed with regional loss of normal autoregulation and can be accompanied by superimposed ischemia. The initiation of swelling results from cerebral vasodilatation followed by a breakdown of the blood brain barrier, leading to cerebral edema. Some authorities have suggested that in a patient in whom a SDH is not clinically apparent until 2–3 days after the injury, the progressive development of brain swelling is more likely the cause of clinical deterioration and elevated ICP than hematoma expansion.

Diffuse swelling of both cerebral hemispheres tends to occur in young patients. The pathogenesis of this type of brain damage is unclear, but in the pediatric population, dysfunctional autoregulation leading to a loss of vasomotor tone and consequent vasodilatation may contribute to the swelling. If the vasodilatation persists, the blood brain barrier may become defective and true edema may result.

Superimposed ischemic and hypoxic brain damage is common in patients that sustain severe blunt traumatic head injury. It is significantly more common in patients who sustain a clinical episode of hypotension or hypoxia (systolic blood pressure (SBP) <80 mmHg for at least 15 min, or a PaO_2 <50 mmHg at some time after injury) than in those who do not. Such damage is also more common in patients who experience high ICPs. A significant correlation also exists between ischemic brain damage in patients who sustain blunt head injury and arterial spasm. The presence of ischemic damage in arterial watershed areas suggests that the patient may sustain a period of cerebral perfusion failure due to an episode of hypotension. Ischemic damage is thus another potential cause of traumatic coma in the absence of an intracranial mass lesion. Such damage is also a frequent finding in patients who remain vegetative or severely disabled after sustaining a head injury.

Evaluation and Management of Severe Closed Head Injury

Early clinical recognition and radiographic diagnosis are key initial steps in the management of head injury. Also important is the need for serial clinical and radiographic assessment of the head-injured patient as the primary thrust of management should be geared towards determining whether the patient has a lesion that requires urgent neurosurgical attention. The initial neurologic assessment of a head-injured patient should be prompt and aimed at evaluating the patient's level of consciousness, as well as symmetry of neurologic function from head to toe. This should include a determination of the patient's Glasgow Coma Scale (GCS) score, a cranial nerve exam that evaluates pupillary function, extraocular movements, facial symmetry, and vital cranial nerve reflexes, as well as a good motor exam. A thorough motor examination, however, may be difficult owing to the presence of other systemic injury, other ongoing diagnostic and therapeutic maneuvers, and lack of patient cooperation. The data acquired are an important indicator of the significance and severity of possible cerebral and brainstem compression. In a pharmacologically paralyzed patient, the pupillary exam encompasses the entirety of the neurologic examination and must be performed in an accurate and serial fashion.

A prompt radiographic evaluation with a noncontrast head CT scan should follow the neurologic assessment, but may be delayed depending on the patient's resuscitative needs and the resources of the treating facility. The identification of a mass lesion or significant alteration in GCS should prompt an urgent neurosurgical consultation.

Surgical Management

In 2006, the Congress of Neurologic Surgeons formed guidelines for the surgical management of traumatic brain injury (TBI). The guidelines are briefly summarized as follows:

- EDHs > 30 ml in volume should be surgically evacuated regardless of the patient's GCS score. Patients with an acute EDH in coma (GCS <9) with pupillary asymmetry should undergo surgical evacuation as soon as possible.
- An acute SDH with thickness >10 mm or a midline shift >5 mm on CTscan should be surgically evacuated regardless of GCS score. All patients with acute SDH in coma should undergo ICP monitoring. A comatose patient with an SDH <10 mm thickness and a midline shift <5 mm should undergo surgical evacuation if the GCS score decreases between the time of injury and hospital admission by two or more points, and/or the patient presents with asymmetric or fixed and dilated pupils, and/or the ICP exceeds 20 mmHg.
- Patients with parenchymal mass lesions (contusions and intracerebral hematomas) and signs of progressive

neurological deterioration referable to the lesion, medically refractory intracranial hypertension, or signs of mass effect on CT scan should be treated operatively. Patients' GCS scores of 6–8 with frontal or temporal lesions <20 ml in volume with a midline shift of at least 5 mm and/or cisternal compression on CT scan, and patients with any lesion >50 cc in volume should be treated operatively.

Medical Management

In the absence of a surgical lesion, rapid and aggressive medical management should be instituted. The medical management of the head-injured patient is directed largely at supportive therapy, as well as the prevention and treatment of the secondary effects of traumatic head injury which manifest primarily as raised ICP.

We tend to err on the side of initiating aggressive treatment of patients with presumed severe TBI (GCS <8) before a radiographic diagnosis is made because we believe that the rapid initiation of therapeutic measures is paramount in preventing insults that may result from the secondary effects of traumatic head injury. Our treatment strategy is based largely on guidelines set forth by the Brain Trauma Foundation and Joint Section on Neurotrauma and Critical Care of the AANS in 2000 entitled Management and Prognosis of Severe Traumatic Brain Injury, and is summarized below. While much of this summary comes directly from these guidelines, we have indicated our favored management approaches wherever appropriate.

General Care and Supportive Measures

Hypotension (SBP <90 mmHg) and hypoxia (apnea, cyanosis, and oxygen (O_2) saturation <90% in the field or a PaO_2 <60 mmHg) must be monitored, and avoided if possible or corrected immediately in severe TBI patients. The mean arterial pressure (MAP) should be maintained above 90 mmHg through the infusion of fluids, and judicious use of vasopressors if necessary. Patients who are unable to maintain their airway or remain hypoxemic despite supplemental O_2, must have their airway secured, preferably by endotracheal intubation. Central venous pressure and invasive blood pressure monitoring are mandatory. A Swan-Ganz catheter should be considered strongly in patients with cardiopulmonary disease or those requiring extensive vasopressor therapy. Red blood cell rheology, as well as the oxygen-carrying capacity of blood, should be optimized by maintaining a hematocrit between 30% and 34%. All efforts should be made to avoid hyperglycemia as this can be common in head-injured patients, and may aggravate cerebral edema and secondary injury. Strict glycemic control with frequent blood glucose checks and treatment of elevated levels (<150 mg/dl) with subcutaneous or IV insulin is strongly encouraged. As a treatment option, anticonvulsants may be used to prevent early post-traumatic seizures (seizures occurring within 7 days of the initial injury) in patients at high risk for seizures following head injury. Prophylactic therapy should last no longer than 7 days. Phenytoin and carbamazepine have been shown to be effective in preventing early post-traumatic seizures. However, there is not sufficient evidence to demonstrate that the prevention of early post-traumatic seizures improves outcome following head injury. The use of steroids is not recommended for improving outcome or reducing ICP in patients with severe TBI, as it has not been shown to improve outcome and results in increased complication rates.

Intracranial Pressure Monitoring

ICP monitoring is appropriate in patients with GCS scores of 3–8 after adequate cardiopulmonary resuscitation and abnormal head CT that reveals hematomas, edema, contusions, or compressed basal cisterns. It is appropriate in patients with GCS scores of 3–8 with normal head CT if two or more of the following are noted on admission: age >40 years, unilateral or bilateral posturing, SBP <90 mmHg. It is not routinely indicated in patients with mild (GCS 13–15) to moderate (GCS 9–12) head injury; however, a physician may choose to monitor ICP in certain conscious patients with traumatic mass lesions. In the current state of technology, the ventricular catheter connected to an external strain gauge is the most accurate, low-cost, and reliable method of monitoring ICP. It also allows therapeutic CSF drainage. Parenchymal ICP monitoring is similar to ventricular ICP monitoring, but has the potential for measurement drift. Subarachnoid, subdural, and epidural monitors are currently less accurate. The authors' monitor of choice is the ventricular catheter for reasons expressed above. However, in patients with small ventricles, we elect to place a parenchymal monitor if attempts at ventricular cannulation are unsuccessful.

Management of Elevated Intracranial Pressure

Elevations in ICP are tolerated poorly in head injury patients compared with normal individuals because of concomitant dysfunctional autoregulation, brain swelling, and underlying hypoxic ischemic damage (Table 9.1). The intracranial cavity consists of CSF, blood, and brain parenchyma. Following head injury, several mechanisms are set in motion in an attempt to counteract ICP elevations in accordance with the Monroe-Kellie doctrine. Initially, CSF volume is reduced by displacement of CSF from the intracranial to the spinal compartment, as well as increased CSF resorption. Continued increases in ICP are compensated for by decreases in the intracranial volume by venous compression. If the ICP continues to rise, however, compensatory mechanisms are exhausted, intracranial compliance decreases, and, as a result, smaller changes in volume lead to larger elevations of ICP. ICP treatment should be initiated at an upper threshold of 20 mmHg. Interpretation and treatment of ICP based on any threshold should be corroborated by frequent clinical examination and cerebral perfusion pressure (CPP) data, which is determined by calculating the

TABLE 9.1. Outline of management strategy to treat elevated ICP.

First-line therapy	*Positional changes*
	Maintain head of bed at 30–45°
	Keep neck straight
	Avoid constrictive devices about cervical spine
	Control PaCO$_2$
	Mild hyperventilation (maintain PaCO$_2$ between 30–35 mmHg)
	Hyperosmolar therapy
	Mannitol
	Hypertonic saline
	Sedation
	Diprivan (Propofol)
	Lorazepam (Ativan)
	Midazolam (Versed)
	Chemical paralysis
Second-line therapy	*Aggressive hyperventilation* (maintain PaCO$_2$ < 30 mmHg; short duration only)
	High-dose barbiturate therapy
	Decompressive craniectomy

difference between the MAP and the ICP. CPP should be maintained at a minimum of 60 mmHg. It remains a crude but rapid estimation of blood flow to the brain. If available, more sophisticated determinants of cerebral blood flow (CBF) may be employed. It is important to note that ICP elevations above 20 mmHg are more deleterious to head trauma patients than decreases in CPP below 60 mmHg, and higher CPPs are not as protective in patients with elevated ICPs. Thus every effort should be made to keep the ICP below 20 mmHg.

Elevations in ICP are initially treated with elevation of the patient's head to 30°, mild hyperventilation maintaining the PaCO2 between 30 and 35 mmHg, CSF drainage, hyperosmolar therapy with mannitol or 3% sodium chloride, sedation with diprivan (Propofol), lorezapam (Ativan), midazolam (Versed) and/or morphine, and chemical paralysis. The elevation of the patient's head of bed up to 30–45° while keeping the neck straight and avoiding any constricting devices around the cervical region, helps facilitate venous drainage without compromising the arterial blood supply. Mild hyperventilation results in a decrease in $PaCO_2$, which ultimately leads to cerebral vasoconstriction and a decrease in CBF followed by a decrease in ICP. Mild hyperventilation therapy ($PaCO_2$ between 30 and 35 mmHg) may be useful during long periods of refractory intracranial hypertension. In the presence of increased ICPs, prolonged aggressive hyperventilation therapy ($PaCO_2 < 25$ mmHg) should be avoided in severe TBI given its effects on cerebral perfusion and potential for cerebral ischemia, especially in the first 24 h following injury when cerebral blood flows. For the same reason, prophylactic hyperventilation therapy should be avoided if possible. However, more aggressive hyperventilation therapy ($PaCO_2$ <30 mmHg) may be necessary for brief periods when there is acute neurologic deterioration.

Mannitol is effective for control of raised ICP after severe TBI. Effective doses range from 0.25 to 1 g/kg body weight. The indications for use of mannitol prior to ICP monitoring are signs of transtentorial herniation or progressive neurologic deterioration not attributable to extracranial complaints. The patient's fluid status must be monitored closely, especially when there is concomitant use of diuretics to ensure the avoidance of hypovolemia and hypotension. Mannitol increases the osmolality of blood acutely, which helps withdraw water from the brain into the bloodstream. It is effective only with an intact blood brain barrier, however, and a delayed rebound phenomenon of elevated ICP can occur secondary to the entry of mannitol into the brain. It also functions as a free radical scavenger and decreases blood viscosity, which transiently increases CBF and triggers cerebral vasoconstriction, which in turn acutely lowers ICP. Serum osmolarity should be kept below 320 mOsm due to concerns for renal failure. Intermittent boluses may be more effective than a continuous infusion of mannitol. Hypertonic saline (3% or 7.5% NaCl; some investigators use even higher concentrations) is an accepted alternative to mannitol. Like mannitol, it is effective in treating elevated ICP, and has favorable effects of cerebral perfusion and red blood cell rheology. However, it has a more favorable side-effect profile and is the authors' preferred choice for hyperosmolar therapy in the setting of prolonged (>3–5 days) intracranial hypertension.

Precipitous spikes in ICP should be evaluated with a noncontrast head CT scan. This is aimed at detecting a surgical lesion before it contributes to refractory intracranial hypertension.

"Second-Line" Therapy for Persistent Elevated Intracranial Pressure

In the event that the above-described measures are unsuccessful in addressing elevated ICPs, "second-line" therapy may be instituted. These measures are so named because they are either effective therapies with significant risks or are unproven in terms of benefit on outcome. They include aggressive hyperventilation, high-dose barbiturate therapy, hypothermia, and decompressive craniectomy.

High-dose barbiturate therapy may be considered in hemodynamically salvageable, severe TBI patients with intracranial hypertension refractory to maximum medical and surgical ICP-lowering therapy. The benefits of barbiturates stem from vasoconstriction in normal areas (shunting blood to ischemic brain tissue), decreased metabolic demand for oxygen (CMRO2) with accompanying reduction of CBF, free radical scavenging, reduced intracellular calcium, and lysosomal stabilization. The primary side effect is hypotension due to barbiturate-induced direct myocardial depression and reduction of sympathetic tone, which leads to peripheral vasodilatation.

Induced hypothermia carries many systemic side effects including pneumonia, thrombocytopenia, pancreatitis, renal failure, and myocardial depression. Whole-body temperature reductions are slowly giving way to focal cerebral hypothermia, which appears to have a lower side-effect profile.

Decompressive craniectomy involves the removal of a portion of the calvaria with or without the resection of large areas of contused brain. This measure remains controversial, as results of clinical studies to date have been inconsistent and remain under investigation.

Selected Readings

Bullock MR, et al. (2000) Guidelines for the management of severe traumatic brain injury. American Association of Neurologic Surgeons, Joint Section on Neurotrauma and Critical Care & Traumatic Brain Trauma Foundation, New York

Bullock MR, et al. (2006) Guidelines for the surgical management of traumatic brain injury. Neurosurgery 58(Suppl 3):S2–vi

Lyons MK, Meyer FB (1990) Cerebrospinal fluid physiology and the management of increased intracranial pressure. Mayo Clinic Proc 65:684–707

Rea GL, Rockwold GL (1983) Barbiturate therapy in uncontrolled intracranial hypertension. Neurosurgery; 12:401–404

Tindall GT, Cooper PR, Barrow DL (1996) The practice of neurosurgery, Vol 2. William & Wilkins, Baltimore, MD, pp 1385–1425

Wilkins RH, Rengachary SS (eds) (1996) Neurosurgery, 2nd edn 3 vols. McGraw-Hill, New York, pp 2624–2634

10

Pericardial Tamponade

Gary A. Vercruysse, S. Rob Todd, and Frederick A. Moore

Pearls and Pitfalls

- All wounds between the nipples along the length of the sternum have potential to cause pericardial tamponade.
- Treat all potential intrapericardial injuries as an emergency.
- The Focused Assessment for the Sonographic Examination of the Trauma Patient (FAST) is an excellent tool for diagnosis of pericardial effusion.
- Pericardiocentesis is now less often necessary in a trauma center.
- Clamshell Thoracotomy will decompress both a tension pneumothorax and pericardial tamponade.
- A pericardial window should rarely, if ever, be done outside the operating room.
- A pericardial window is easiest to perform through the midline, tendinous portion of the diaphragm.
- If the abdomen is open, cardiac access is easiest through a median sternotomy.
- If the abdomen is closed, and the patient is in extremis, cardiac access is easiest through a clamshell thoracotomy.

K.I. Bland et al. (eds.), *Trauma Surgery*,
DOI 10.1007/978-1-84996-375-6_10,
© Springer-Verlag London Limited 2011

Introduction

Life-threatening pericardial tamponade is seen most commonly after penetrating trauma, and occasionally after blunt trauma. Chronic medical conditions may also lead to this phenomenon. Survival is greater in those sustaining knife rather than missile wounds. This observation is intuitive, given the fact that gunshot wounds cause cavitary injury as well as direct injury. Anatomically speaking, atrial injuries are more survivable than ventricular injuries. The low pressure atrium tends to bleed less rapidly than the ventricle, and thus does not lead to rapid, high volume accumulation of pericardial blood. The resulting low pressure tamponade is difficult to diagnose and may not manifest until aggressive volume loading increases accumulation of blood within the pericardium. This chapter will focus on traumatic pericardial tamponade. Specifically, we will discuss its pathophysiology and clinical presentations, diagnostic modalities, and management options.

Pathophysiology and Clinical Presentation

Pericardial tamponade is categorized into two phases: well compensated and poorly compensated. Initially when a patient suffers an injury that leads to pericardial tamponade, the heart chambers are being compressed by blood collecting within the relatively nondistendable pericardium. Volume-loading augments cardiac preload; thus an increase in cardiac filling pressures and resultant increase in Starling forces allow cardiac output to be maintained. This situation represents well-compensated pericardial tamponade. In contrast, as pressure around the heart increases because of ongoing bleeding into the pericardium, preload cannot compensate for the added pressure, and cardiac output suffers. This situation is poorly compensated tamponade and is characterized by tachycardia and a narrowed pulse pressure. The time frame during which this progression occurs is variable, and depends on numerous factors, including underlying medical conditions, cardiac reserve, and the extent of the injury.

Pericardial tamponade after trauma can be seen immediately, as with penetrating injuries to the heart or great vessels, or may present in a delayed fashion. Typically, the delayed presentation is seen days to weeks after the inciting injury. Delayed presentation of pericardial tamponade may occur do to eventual rupture of an injured atrial or ventricular wall, with perforation occurring at the site of a focal contusion. More often, delayed presentation of pericardial tamponade occurs without cardiac rupture. Typically, these patients have suffered blunt chest trauma and may have been coagulopathic at the time of presentation. Presumably, a small amount of blood from a myocardial contusion allows for the gradual exudative accumulation of fluid with pericardium. An alternate cause is the post-cardiac injury syndrome, which is associated with fever and either a pleural or pericardial effusion.

Diagnosis

Clinical

Classically, Beck's triad is used to describe pericardial tamponade. This triad consists of distended neck veins, muffled heart sounds, and hypotension. In the best of circumstances it is only seen in about 25% of patients; however, we acknowledge that in a noisy trauma bay, Beck's triad is identified rarely. Were an electrocardiogram to be performed at this point, it would be of relatively low voltage compared with normal. As intrapericardial pressure increases, diastolic volume decreases, and a compensatory tachycardia occurs, allowing for maintenance of cardiac output. As more fluid accumulates around the heart, tamponade becomes critical, and equalization of atrial and ventricular pressures occurs. Pulses paradoxus, another phenomenon seen in pericardial tamponade, is the decrease of arterial pressure by 10 mmHg or greater during inspiration. This finding is seen in critical tamponade when a marked shift of the ventricular septum into the left ventricle as right heart filling occurs with inspiration, which leads to a decrease in left ventricular end-diastolic volume and stroke volume. Eventually, as diastolic filling time becomes shortened, myocardial perfusion is compromised, and subendocardial ischemia and a lethal arrhythmia lead to sudden death.

Chest Radiograph

The typical, portable, recumbent trauma chest radiograph is suggestive of pericardial tamponade to varying degrees, depending on the degree of tamponade present at the time the film is acquired. These films are more sensitive in detecting rib or sternal fractures, tension pneumothorax, and tension hemothorax, but these chest radiographs can be useful tools nonetheless. A trauma radiograph typical of massive pericardial tamponade is shown in Fig. 10.1. If time permits, diagnosis of tamponade

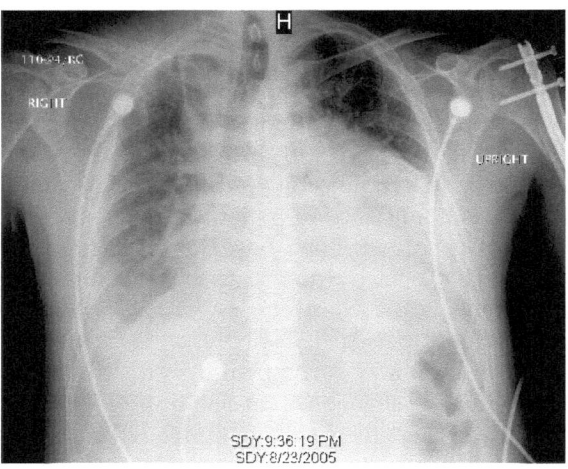

FIGURE 10.1. A chest radiograph typical of that seen with massive pericardial tamponade. Notice the shifted trachea and very enlarged cardiac silhouette.

should be correlated with ultrasonography, or physical signs and symptoms prior to undergoing pericardiocentesis or pericardial window, because a large heart can confuse the picture and lead to unnecessary and at times harmful procedures.

FAST Examination

The (FAST) examination is used to diagnose rapidly the presence of free intra abdominal and pericardial fluid. It is used classically in situations of hemodynamic instability after blunt trauma. The FAST examination has four windows, one of which is the pericardial window. This window is sensitive for the detection of intrapericardial fluid and has become very useful in the workup of both blunt and penetrating trauma. The examination can be done with portable equipment in only a couple of minutes and yields very important data. In a classic paper by Rozycki and colleagues in Atlanta, the accuracy of the pericardial view of the FAST examination was studied in patients with truncal trauma without an immediate indication for operative intervention. Of 247 patients examined, 236 FAST exams were true negative examinations, and 10 were true positive examinations. There were no false negative or false positive examinations. Mean duration of the examination was 48 s. The mean time from FAST exam to operation was 12.1 min, and there were no related mortalities. A positive exam is based on three findings: (1) separation of the pericardial layers with an anechoic area, (2) a decrease in the motion of the parietal pericardium, and (3) identification of the swinging motion of the heart within the pericardial sac. It is important to note that this examination is not static and depends on visualizing both the lack of motion of the pericardium and the extra motion of the "ballotable" heart within the pericardium. An example of a positive pericardial window is seen in > Fig. 10.2. Although this study was done at an institution where FAST has become second nature to those performing the exam, with adequate training and practice, this is the easiest and least invasive maneuver for diagnosing pericardial tamponade.

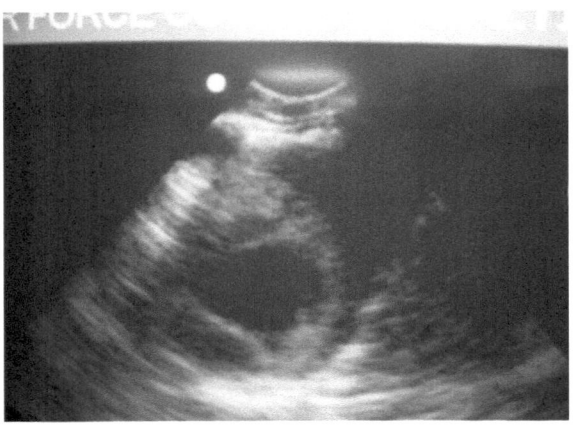

FIGURE 10.2. FAST examination showing a positive pericardial view.

Computed Tomography

Computed tomography (CT) is becoming ever more useful to the trauma surgeon in the evaluation of stable trauma patients. With the advent of multi detector, helical, CT, a full body scan can be completed in only a few minutes. It should be stressed however, the hemodynamically unstable patient is not a candidate for CT. Occasionally, delayed pericardial tamponade can be diagnosed with CT. Fig. 10.3 depicts one such example. This patient required endotracheal intubation for respiratory distress 15 days after bilateral long bone and pelvic fractures, as well as multiple rib fractures and pulmonary contusion. He underwent thoracic CT-angiography to exclude pulmonary embolus. Cardiac tamponade was diagnosed, and he was taken to the operating suite immediately for a pericardial window that drained 1.9 l of serosanguineous fluid. This patient was coagulopathic due to a combination of relative malnutrition (vitamin K deficiency) and use of prophylactic low molecular weight heparin, and likely sequestered the fluid secondary to the osmotic load of the old blood and his hypoalbuminemia. He recovered without further sequelae.

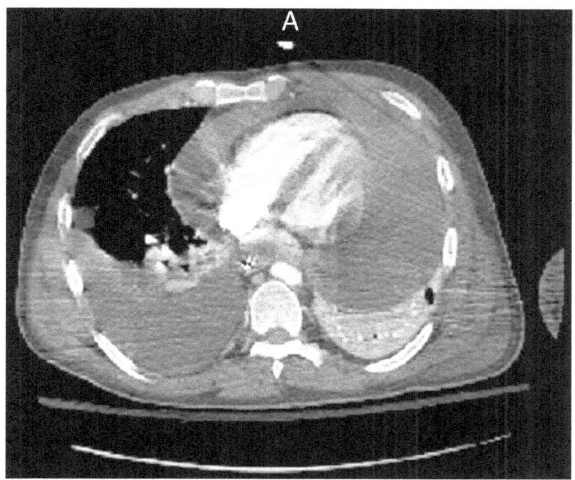

FIGURE 10.3. Computed tomographic image showing massive pericardial tamponade.

Central Venous Catheter

Initial volume loading of the hypotensive trauma patient is standard of care per the Advanced Trauma Life Support course (ATLS). The response to this empiric intervention can help differentiate the type of shock affecting the patient. Patients who respond to fluid loading are most likely hypovolemic, and attention should be directed at identifying the source of bleeding. Patients who do not respond are either in severe hypovolemic shock, cardiogenic shock or neurogenic shock. Because most patients tolerate neurogenic shock, it is imperative to differentiate ongoing hypovolemia from cardiogenic shock.

When inserted while the patient is in the trauma bay, the central venous catheter can be used to help facilitate resuscitation and to diagnose pericardial tamponade. When measuring pressures, a central venous pressure >20 mmHg suggests either tension pneumothorax or, if there is a trend of increasing central venous pressure and decreasing systolic blood pressure, then cardiogenic shock or tamponade. A pressure <5 mmHg suggests hypovolemia.

Pulmonary Artery Catheter

In experienced hands, a pulmonary artery catheter (PAC) is very helpful in the resuscitation of critically ill trauma patient who is not responding to ongoing volume loading. In addition to directing resuscitation, a PAC can be useful in the diagnosis of pericardial tamponade. This mode of diagnosis will most likely be used in the setting of delayed tamponade as these catheters are not normally placed in the trauma bay. A PAC showing increased and equal right atrial, right ventricular end diastolic, and pulmonary artery end diastolic pressures is pathognomonic of pericardial tamponade.

Management

Patients arriving with decompensated pericardial tamponade appear ill and are in obvious distress. In this situation, one needs to avoid the reflex of early intubation as this may precipitate cardiac arrest. These patients are extremely dependent on preload to maintain cardiac filling and are maintaining mean arterial pressure by intense vasoconstriction. Pharmacologic agents used in intubation cause vasodilatation and positive airway pressure decreases preload. The combination can precipitate sudden and fatal pulseless electrical activity.

In penetrating thoraco-abdominal trauma, while the airway is assessed and vascular access is obtained, a chest radiograph and FAST examination are both essential in ruling out not only pericardial tamponade but also hemopneumothoraces. If the patient is hypotensive or extremely tachycardiac, and a positive pericardial view is obtained on FAST examination, a pericardiocentesis may be performed to drain temporarily the pericardium. When performing pericardiocentesis, if a central line kit is used, a catheter may be left in the pericardial space to facilitate further drainage while quickly transporting the patient to the operating room. This is the only situation in which we advocate pericardiocentesis.

If the patient is stable and has a positive pericardial view, time should not be spent performing a pericardiocentesis as this may do more harm than good. The best option in this situation is a controlled subxyphoid pericardial window performed in an expectant manner, in a sterile environment where the equipment necessary for cardiac and/or major vascular repair is located. As long as the patient is stable, pericardial window should not be attempted in the trauma bay, as a positive window leads inevitably to median sternotomy and major vascular or cardiac repair, neither of which can be facilitated in this location. After transport to the operating room, the patient should be prepped and draped prior to the induction of general anesthesia, because positive pressure ventilation, vasodilatory drugs, and the cardio-depressant effects of anesthesia may lead to acute decompensation and cardiovascular collapse on induction. If the patient is in the operating room for another reason and celiotomy has already been performed, pericardial window is easiest through the central tendinous portion of the diaphragm and can be accomplished in a matter of seconds and repaired just as quickly.

If the patient is in extremis, a clamshell thoracotomy will facilitate both emergency drainage of the pericardial sac, clamping of the descending aorta if necessary, and cardiopulmonary resuscitation. Cardiac or great vessel injuries will require temporizing measures, often necessitating finger tamponade while moving the patient to a sterile environment with adequate anesthesia support, instrumentation, and lighting for definitive repair (i.e., the operating room); attempts at definitive repair in the trauma bay delay effective repair and are fraught with complications.

Cases of blunt trauma with evidence of immediate pericardial tamponade should be managed in a manner identical to that for penetrating trauma. In these instances, the patient has likely suffered cardiac rupture. For most patients with delayed pericardial tamponade without cardiac rupture, treatment is a subxyphoid pericardial window with closed tube drainage. Less invasive modalities or pericardiocentesis with catheter drainage may also be employed in this situation.

Asystole in the Field

This problem involves a subset of patients in which pericardial tamponade may occur and immediate intervention may be life-saving. In the case of lost vital signs in the field, the question has been raised repeatedly as to whether or not emergency department (ED) thoracotomy is indicated. A recent study by Moore and colleagues out of Denver found that if a penetrating trauma victim lost vital signs for less than 15 min or a blunt trauma victim for less than 5 min, immediate ED thoracotomy can be life-saving. In their study, five of the patients were in asystole (narrow complex pulseless electrical activity) at the time of ED thoracotomy, all had pericardial tamponade from ventricular stab wounds, four of the five patients had good neurologic outcomes. Unfortunately, in their study, outcomes in victims of blunt trauma were uniformly bad. Although they had no functional survivors in their blunt trauma cohort, they recommend ED thoracotomy for patients who received cardiopulmonary resuscitation (CPR) for less than 5 min given the fact that case reports are published showing satisfactory outcomes in patients who loose vital signs immediately prior to ED arrival.

Summary

Pericardial tamponade is a surgical emergency. In the field of trauma surgery, many patients will die prior to arrival at the trauma center secondary to acute tamponade. Both physical examination and chest radiography may suggest tamponade. The FAST examination in combination with a good physical examination and chest radiograph is diagnostic in the majority of patients with cardiac tamponade. Pericardial window and ultimately cardiorrhaphy or vascular repair can be lifesaving. When evaluating a trauma patient, do not lose sight of the basics. Diagnosis of pericardial tamponade is not a diagnostic tour de force, but delay in its treatment may have lethal consequences.

Selected Readings

Gabram S, Devanney J, Jones D, et al. (1992) Delayed hemorrhagic pericardial effusion: case reports of a complication from severe blunt chest trauma. J Trauma 32:794–800

Mangram A, Kozar R, Gregoric I, et al. (2003) Blunt cardiac injuries that require operative intervention: an unsuspected injury. J Trauma 54:286–288

Powell DW, Moore EE, Cothren CC, et al. (2004) Is emergency department resuscitative thoracotomy futile care for the critically injured patient requiring prehospital cardiopulmonary resuscitation? J Am Coll Surg 199:211–215

Rozycki GS, Feliciano DV, Schmidt JA, et al. (1996) The role of surgeon-performed ultrasound in patients with possible cardiac wounds. Ann Surg 223:737–746

Solomon D (1991) Delayed cardiac tamponade after blunt chest trauma: case report. J Trauma 31:1322–1324

Index

A

Abdomen, 33–47
Abdominal compartment
	syndrome (ACS), 121–135
Abdominal trauma, 19–31
Acute burn surgery, 77
Airway control, 1, 4, 10

B

Blunt, 50, 52, 53, 56, 58–62
Blunt head injury, 138–146
Blunt trauma, 19–31
Brain injury, 137–154
Burn, 67–77, 79, 80
Burn resuscitation, 67–69, 77, 80
Burn size determination, 74

C

Cerebral edema, 83, 85, 98
Cerebral perfusion pressure
	(CPP), 150, 151
Chest, 33, 38–41, 43, 45
Chest trauma, 157, 158
Closed head injury, 83–101
Computed tomography (CT), 19,
	23–26, 30
CPP. See Cerebral perfusion
	pressure
Critical illness, 128

D

DAI. See Diffuse axonal injury
Damage control, 42, 44–47,
	57, 61
Decompression, 103, 104, 107,
	112–118
Depressed skull fractures,
	138–140
Diagnosis of burn depth, 74
Diagnostic peritoneal lavage
	(DPL), 19, 20, 23, 25–27, 30
Diagnostics, 121, 124, 134
Diffuse axonal injury (DAI), 137,
	143–145

E

Epidural hematomas (EDH),
	139–142, 147
Extremity, 49–65

F

Focused abdominal sonography
	for trauma (FAST), 19, 20,
	23–26, 30

G

Glasgow Coma Scale (GCS), 138,
	146–150

H
Heart injury, 156, 157
Hemorrhage, 49–51, 55, 56, 58, 62
High-energy trauma, 19, 20, 29
Hypotension, 157, 161, 162

I
Injury, 49–65
Intra-abdominal hypertension
     (IAH), 121, 123–125, 127,
     132, 134
Intra-abdominal pressure (IAP),
     121–124, 126–133
Intracranial pressure (ICP), 83,
     92–94, 97, 98
Intracranial pressure monitoring,
     147, 149–150, 152

M
Management, 132–134
Moribund trauma, 27–28
Multiple trauma, 20, 21

N
Neck, 33–47
Neuroinflammation, 83, 93
Neuropharmacology,

O
Outcome of burn victims, 80

P
Pathophysiology, 127, 133
Penetrating, 33–47, 50, 51, 55, 56,
     58–60, 62
Penetrating head injury, 138–140

Pericardial tamponade, 155–164
Primary survey, 2–14, 16, 17

R
Reduction, 103–105, 110, 112–116,
     119
Rehabilitation, 105, 118

S
SDH. *See* Subdural hematomas
Secondary survey, 3, 12–18
Shock, 2, 6–8, 12, 161
Spinal cord injury (SCI), 103–106,
     117, 118
Spine, 103–119
Stabilization, 103, 104, 109, 112,
     113, 115, 116, 119
Subdural hematomas (SDH),
     139–143, 145, 147
Surgery, 103, 113–114, 116–119

T
Therapy, 132
Thoracoabdominal, 49–65
Trauma, 1–18, 49–65, 103–119
Traumatic brain injury, 84
Treatment of burn wounds,
     76–80

U
Ultrasonography (US), 19, 23–24
Unstable, 27, 28

V
Vascular, 49–65
Vessel, 50, 52, 53, 55, 58–62, 64